Using Human Factors Engineering to Improve Patient Safety:
Problem Solving on the Front Line

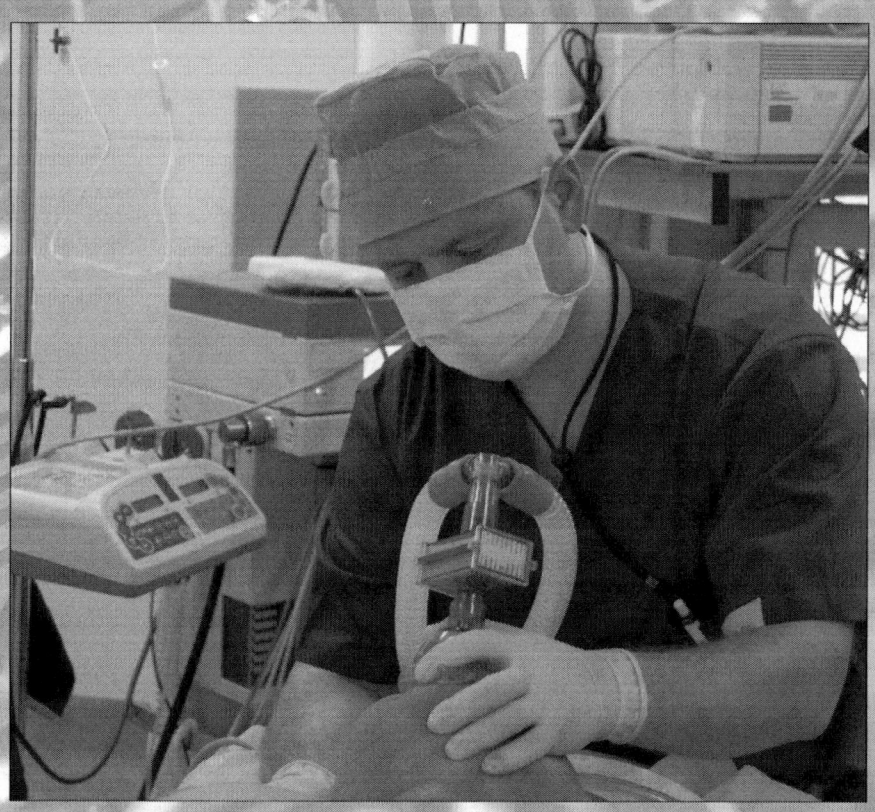

SECOND EDITION

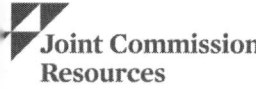
Joint Commission Resources

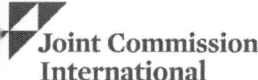
Joint Commission International

Editors
John W. Gosbee, M.D., M.S.
Laura Lin Gosbee, M.A.Sc.

USING HUMAN FACTORS ENGINEERING TO IMPROVE PATIENT SAFETY:
Problem Solving on the Front Line | Second Edition

Executive Editor: Steven Berman
Senior Project Manager: Cheryl Firestone
Manager, Publications: Paul Reis
Associate Director, Production: Johanna Harris
Executive Director: Catherine Chopp Hinckley, Ph.D.
Joint Commission/JCR Reviewers: Pat Adamski, Gerry Castro, Nanne Finis, Catherine Chopp Hinckley, Rick Morrow, Paul Reis, Heather Sherman

Joint Commission Resources Mission
The mission of Joint Commission Resources (JCR) is to continuously improve the safety and quality of care in the United States and in the international community through the provision of education and consultation services and international accreditation.

Joint Commission International
A division of Joint Commission Resources, Inc.
The mission of Joint Commission International (JCI) is to improve the safety and quality of care in the international community through the provision of education, publications, consultation, and evaluation services.

Joint Commission Resources educational programs and publications support, but are separate from, the accreditation activities of Joint Commission International. Attendees at Joint Commission Resources educational programs and purchasers of Joint Commission Resources publications receive no special consideration or treatment in, or confidential information about, the accreditation process.

The inclusion of an organization name, product, or service in a Joint Commission Resources publication should not be construed as an endorsement of such organization, product, or services, nor is failure to include an organization name, product, or service to be construed as disapproval.

© 2010 by The Joint Commission

Joint Commission Resources, Inc. (JCR), a not-for-profit affiliate of The Joint Commission, has been designated by The Joint Commission to publish publications and multimedia products. JCR reproduces and distributes these materials under license from the Joint Commission.

All rights reserved. No part of this publication may be reproduced in any form or by any means without written permission from the publisher.

Printed in the U.S.A. 5 4 3 2 1

Requests for permission to make copies of any part of this work should be mailed to
Permissions Editor
Department of Publications
Joint Commission Resources
One Renaissance Boulevard
Oakbrook Terrace, Illinois 60181 U.S.A.
permissions@jcrinc.com

ISBN: 978-1-59940-411-0
Library of Congress Control Number: 2010928353

For more information about Joint Commission Resources, please visit http://www.jcrinc.com.
For more information about Joint Commission International, please visit http://www.jointcommissioninternational.org.

Contents

CONTRIBUTORS iv

INTRODUCTION v

PART I: HUMAN FACTORS ENGINEERING

CHAPTER 1: *Theory and General Principles* 3
Laura Lin Gosbee, M.A.Sc.

CHAPTER 2: *Methods and Tools* 35
Laura Lin Gosbee, M.A.Sc.

CHAPTER 3: *Lessons Learned in Teaching Human Factors Engineering* 55
John W. Gosbee, M.D., M.S.; Laura Lin Gosbee, M.A.Sc.

CHAPTER 4: *Finding and Using Human Factors Engineering Expertise* 67
Laura Lin Gosbee, M.A.Sc.; John W. Gosbee, M.D., M.S.

APPENDIX: *Human Factors Engineering Resources* 71

PART II: CASE STUDIES

INTRODUCTION 79

CHAPTER 5: *How I Learned About Human Factors Engineering* 81
Sandra Coletta

CHAPTER 6: *Human Factors Engineering in Action: Sunnybrook's Patient Safety Service* 89
Edward Etchells, M.D., M.Sc.; Catherine O'Neill, R.N., B.Sc.N.; Jeremy I. Robson Ph.D.;
Richard Mraz, P.Eng; Julie Chan, B.A.Sc., M.H.Sc.; Patti Cornish, B.Sc.Phm.

CHAPTER 7: *Human Factors Engineering at The Johns Hopkins Hospital* 103
Peter A. Doyle, Ph.D.

CHAPTER 8: *Applying Human Factors Engineering in a Patient Safety and Quality Program* 117
Laurie D. Wolf, M.S., C.P.E., A.S.Q.-C.S.S.B.B.

CHAPTER 9: *Integrating Human Factors Engineering Expertise into Patient Safety Research* 135
Yan Xiao, Ph.D.

CHAPTER 10: *Integrating Human Factors Engineering into Medication Safety at ISMP Canada* 145
Sylvia Hyland, R.Ph., B.Sc.Phm., M.H.Sc.; John Senders, Ph.D.

INDEX 157

USING HUMAN FACTORS ENGINEERING TO IMPROVE PATIENT SAFETY:
Problem Solving on the Front Line | Second Edition

Contributors

PART I. HUMAN FACTORS ENGINEERING

Chapters 1–4

John W. Gosbee, M.D., M.S., and **Laura Lin Gosbee, M.A.Sc.,** Human Factors Engineering and Healthcare Specialists, are Principals, Red Forest Consulting, Ann Arbor, Michigan.

PART II. CASE STUDIES

Chapter 5. How I Learned About Human Factors Engineering

Sandra Coletta is President and Chief Executive Officer, Kent Hospital, Warwick, Rhode Island.

Chapter 6. Human Factors Engineering In Action: Sunnybrook's Patient Safety Service

Edward Etchells, M.D., M.Sc., is Associate Director, University of Toronto Centre for Patient Safety; Medical Director of Information Services, Sunnybrook Health Sciences Centre, Toronto; and Associate Professor of Medicine, University of Toronto. **Catherine O'Neill, R.N., B.Sc.N.,** is Director, Quality and Patient Safety, Quinte Health Care, Belleville, Ontario, Canada. **Jeremy I. Robson, Ph.D.,** is Senior Consultant and Team Manager, HumanSystems® Incorporated, Guelph, Ontario, Canada. **Richard Mraz, P.Eng.,** is Project Manager, Information Services, Sunnybrook Health Sciences Centre. **Julie Chan, B.A.Sc., M.H.Sc.,** is Graduate Student, Information Services, Sunnybrook Health Sciences Centre. **Patti Cornish, B.Sc.Phm.,** is Assistant Registrar, Pharmacy Examining Board of Canada, Toronto.

Chapter 7. Human Factors Engineering at The Johns Hopkins Hospital

Peter A. Doyle, Ph.D., is Human Factors Engineer, Clinical Engineering Services, The Johns Hopkins Hospital, Baltimore.

Chapter 8. Applying Human Factors Engineering in a Patient Safety and Quality Program

Laurie D. Wolf, M.S., C.P.E., A.S.Q.-C.S.S.B.B., is Management Engineer, Operational Excellence Department, Barnes-Jewish Hospital, Edwardsville, Illinois.

Chapter 9. Integrating Human Factors Engineering Expertise into Patient Safety Research

Yan Xiao, Ph.D., is Director of Patient Safety Research, Baylor Health Care System, Dallas.

Chapter 10. Integrating Human Factors Engineering into Medication Safety at ISMP Canada

Sylvia Hyland, R.Ph., M.H.Sc., B.Sc.Phm., is Vice President and Chief Operating Officer, Institute for Safe Medication Practices Canada, Toronto. **John W. Senders, Ph.D.,** is Consulting Scientist; Professor Emeritus, University of Toronto; and Member, Board of Trustees, Institute for Safe Medication Practices Canada.

Introduction

WHY HFE?

If you've heard about human factors engineering (HFE), it may have been in the context of making things "easy to use" or "user friendly." Although these attributes are desirable, it may not be so obvious that the concept of making things "user friendly" can be extended to make a hospital or other health care organization safer and more efficient. HFE is the discipline concerned with understanding human characteristics and applying that knowledge to the design of systems that are reliable, safe, efficient, and comfortable to use (*system* refers to all the elements that are part of the delivery of care to patients).

What makes HFE so valuable is that it attempts to address complexity, something that is abundant in health care. To achieve simplicity of use, safety, and efficiency, HFE uses knowledge of human cognitive and physical capabilities and limitations to design or redesign the tools, tasks, and work areas in health care. HFE complements other quality and patient safety improvement methods that because of their lack of focus on systems design, may lead to solutions that are either inappropriate to the level of complexity, impractical, or inefficient, resulting in workarounds (that is, alternative work procedures undertaken to bypass perceived or real barriers in work flow). According to the HFE perspective, you design the system to fit the human, not the other way around. In so doing, you can create enduring conditions that make it easier for people to reliably carry out work correctly and efficiently. We can alter our tools and work environment, but it is quite difficult, even one can argue, impossible, to alter human nature.

To tackle the formidable challenge of taming complexity, HFE draws upon a broad knowledge base of applied research in human performance. This gives the HFE professional—usually, someone with an human factors degree from a university program, such as engineering or psychology, or even education or computer science (Chapter 4)—an understanding of how and why people interact the way they do with the systems around them. For example, the manner in which people perceive, recall things from memory, or make decisions can determine how easy or difficult it is to program a pump or use an electronic order entry system. In addition, the task at hand imposes its own needs and requirements. If a system does not meet these needs or does so in a clumsy fashion, then it places a mental or physical burden on the person. A system, say, an electronic health record software, might be considered clumsy if, for example, it required the clinician to memorize data from one screen and keep it in memory as he or she navigates to find another screen to enter the data. Alternatively, it may use terminology that is somewhat ambiguous or too technical for the typical clinician. Having frequently used functions buried deep in a menu system is another example of a "clumsy" software system. In all cases, the system does not provide a good fit to either the task or the human.

HFE professionals use a variety of methods and tools to (1) analyze system usability or safety, (2) design solutions, and (3) test the system or solution to determine its impact on human performance.

USING HUMAN FACTORS ENGINEERING TO IMPROVE PATIENT SAFETY:
Problem Solving on the Front Line | Second Edition

PURPOSE OF THIS BOOK

This book, *Using Human Factors Engineering to Improve Patient Safety: Problem Solving on the Front Line,* Second Edition, (1) shows health care organizations how they can develop and use HFE expertise to improve patient safety, and (2) shows HFE professionals how others have pursued a career path to help health care organizations address a variety of HFE–related issues. This twofold purpose is designed to help managers, leaders, and clinicians at health care organizations, and HFE professionals, learn how to work together to best deploy HFE in clinical settings.

NEW IN THIS EDITION

Using Human Factors Engineering to Improve Patient Safety: Problem Solving on the Front Line, Second Edition, like its predecessor, *Using Human Factors Engineering to Improve Patient Safety,* consists of two parts. For Part I, Chapters 1–2 are updated and expanded, and Chapters 3–4 are new. For Part II (Chapters 5–10) in this new edition, we enlisted top experts in the United States and Canada to tell their own stories of how their organizations are deploying HFE to improve patient safety.

OVERVIEW OF CONTENT

Part I

Part I provides basic background on key HFE principles and theories (Chapter 1), which can help you identify systems in your health care organization that are plagued with human factors problems. Chapter 2 guides you through methods and tools that HFE professionals employ in devising solutions. Organizations interested in integrating HFE into their safety and quality activities can learn from step-by-step recommendations provided in Chapters 3 and 4.

Chapter 1 "Theory and General Principles" explores human capabilities and limitations, which will help you recognize the signs and symptoms of human factors issues. This chapter provides readers a basic understanding of how design can either accommodate these human characteristics (good design) or ignore them (poor design).

Chapter 2 "Methods and Tools" discusses the process and methods for diagnosing HFE issues behind adverse events in your health care organization.

Chapter 3 "Lessons Learned in Teaching Human Factors Engineering" reviews the reasons you have missed many design problems "hiding in plain sight" in your setting and provides the "top 10" pearls that we have found useful for the "practice" of HFE.

Chapter 4 "Finding and Using Human Factors Engineering Expertise" includes "Finding the HFE Professional 'Right' for the Organization" which provides tips and recommendations for health care organizations that want to recruit HFE professionals and integrate HFE into their quality and patient safety activities. The chapter also highlights the lessons learned from the experiences of the organizations represented in Part II.

Part II

The case-study chapters (Chapters 5–10) provide stories from the front lines of how health care organizations have integrated HFE into their quality and patient safety activities. The chapters provide detailed project-specific accounts of the deployment of HFE principles, theories, and tools described in Chapters 1–2. The projects chosen are not necessarily large but were selected as most representative of the work that HFE professionals conduct on a daily basis to have an impact on patient safety—and, in some cases, efficiency. The Appendix provides references to guidelines, handbooks, HFE textbooks, and special topics for those looking for additional material on HFE.

A NOTE ON TERMINOLOGY

As discussed in Chapter 1, there is considerable diversity in the terminology used to describe HFE, just as there are many paths to becoming an HFE professional or to applying HFE to the health care setting, as discussed in Chapter 4. This diversity will also be readily apparent in Chapters 5–10. Yet differences in terminology should be of minimal concern. Whether starting out in injury prevention, as did Laurie Wolf (Chapter 8), or patient safety research, as did Yan Xiao (Chapter 9), HFE professionals share common methods and mind-sets—and a key focus on redesign to improve outcomes.

WHO SHOULD READ THIS BOOK?

Using Human Factors Engineering to Improve Patient Safety: Problem Solving on the Front Line, Second Edition, is intended for anyone interested in reducing errors in health care and improving patient safety, whether you are a chief executive officer, chief operating officer, patient safety officer, physician, nurse, risk manager, performance improvement professional, physician assistant, or engineer. The book is also addressed to the HFE professionals themselves to learn how to contribute their HFE expertise in improving patient safety on the front line. Whether you are a student working toward an HFE graduate degree or an HFE professional considering a change in career focus, this book provides practical guidance.

This book shows how theory and practice are applied to hospitals, ambulatory care, emergency medical services, and outpatient cancer care. Yet HFE methods are adaptable to all health care organizations, which face the challenge of designing patient safety–enhancing systems that are reliable, efficient, and comfortable for clinicians—and patients—to use.

—*John W. Gosbee, M.D., M.S.*
Laura Lin Gosbee, M.A.Sc.

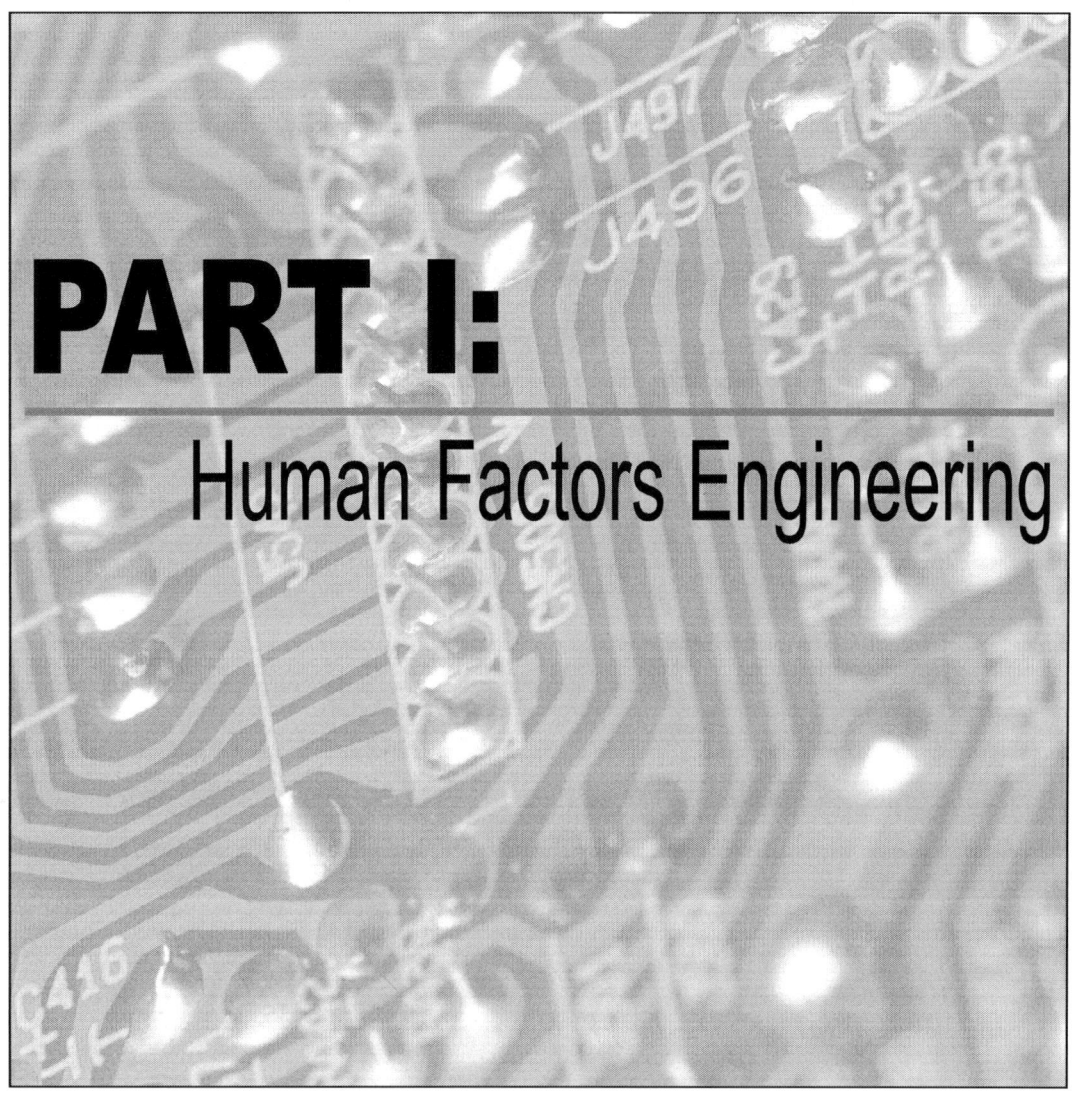

PART I:
Human Factors Engineering

CHAPTER 1

Theory and General Principles

Laura Lin Gosbee, M.A.Sc.

WHY DESIGN MATTERS

Modern advancements in health care technologies have given us remarkable diagnostic and therapeutic capabilities. Operating these technologies and weaving them into existing work environments and tasks can be challenging. Sometimes, highly sophisticated equipment is easy to operate with minimal training. At other times, the interface of the equipment is difficult to understand and use, necessitating extensive training even on how to turn on the equipment. Similar kinds of complexity and inscrutability can also be found in low-technology items such as preprinted order forms, medication labeling, or medication storage areas. Complexity of use, while often associated with advanced technology, is not always a product of technology level.

In some cases, complexity in how a product or device is operated is necessary because its operation requires in-depth knowledge in a particular area of expertise. For example, radiation therapists receive extensive training to operate the sophisticated equipment and computers that are used in the course of radiation treatment for patients with cancer. At other times, the complexity is unnecessary and is the unfortunate (and often unintended) product of engineers or designers focusing their design efforts too narrowly and forgetting about the human operator. An engineer or designer who has spent months, if not years, developing a product may simply lack the perspective to imagine how one could fail to understand how to use it. No matter how technically advanced, the product would be "trapped inside" an interface that can elicit awkward or even dangerous interaction with the human operator.

When the design of a product neglects to take into account the human-interaction dimension, it could lead to undesirable consequences for the operator/user of the product: frustration, delays, tedium, and work-arounds. The end result is not just inefficiency but the circumstances that will make it more likely for errors to occur. A product is only effective, useful, and successful if it is designed such that it can be operated correctly and efficiently.

To the average health care clinician, frustration, tedium, or work-arounds are just part of his or her job. To a human factors engineering (HFE) professional, they are symptoms of ailments deeper in the design of the system, of a misguided focus on technology alone, rather than the human *coupled with* that technology.

HFE is the discipline concerned with understanding human characteristics and applying that knowledge to the design of systems that are reliable, safe, efficient, and comfortable to use. The term *system* is used broadly here to refer to all the elements that are part of the delivery of care to patients. Tools, medical equipment, work-area layout, architecture, tasks, processes, work environment, computer systems, and so on, are all such elements. More specific examples include intravenous (IV) tubing and connectors, monitoring devices, protocols, preprinted order forms, IV pumps, way-finding signs for patients, pathology reports, computer-

> ## Sidebar 1-1. Usability Testing Improves Redesign of Code Cart, Reduces Retrieval Time
>
> One health care facility employed usability testing to help guide its redesign of medication layout in code cart drawers. The facility used results of a series of usability tests to guide how they should refine their design. The result was improved medication retrieval time from an average of 3 min. 7 sec. to 1 min. 8 sec. More details on pages 49–51.
>
> **Source:** McLaughlin R.C.: Redesigning the crash cart: Usability testing improves one facility's medication drawers. *Am J Nurs* 103:64A–64F, Apr. 2003. Used with permission.

ized order entry systems, operating rooms (ORs) and code carts (Sidebar 1-1, above). HFE is often considered synonymous with *ergonomics, human engineering, usability engineering, engineering psychology,* or simply *human factors.* The International Ergonomics Association, a federation of ergonomics and human factors societies from around the world, provides the following definitions:

> Ergonomics (or human factors) is the scientific discipline concerned with the understanding of interactions among humans and other elements of a system, and the profession that applies theory, principles, data and methods to design in order to optimize human well-being and overall system performance. Practitioners of ergonomics (ergonomists) contribute to the planning, design and evaluation of tasks, jobs, products, organizations, environments and systems in order to make them compatible with the needs, abilities and limitations of people.[1]

Adopting an HFE approach to patient safety is needed to overcome the "blame and shame" or "blame and train" attitude. Instead of looking at individuals involved in the adverse event, HFE looks at the *systems failures* behind the event to develop long-lasting solutions. Systems failures—such as a confusing display on a monitor, a tedious programming sequence to set up a pump, a poorly organized storage area, poor lighting, or a poorly structured order set (Sidebar 1-2, page 5)—persist, creating the circumstances for someone else to make an error. Fixing these problems at the source is far more effective at removing the risk of error than to expect humans to adapt, whether it be through training or being more vigilant. The expectation is that, if the conditions (such as the design of the pump, storage area, lighting, and so forth) encourage a certain set of behaviors, then it will be difficult to alter those behaviors without redesigning the conditions that elicited them to begin with.

Health care is following the lead of other high-risk industries, such as aviation and the nuclear power industry, in which attention is placed on the human-system interactions and how the design of systems either encourages or discourages errors. A poorly designed system is one that does not match the needs of the human or task or does not take into account human limitations. Human perception, human memory, and anthropometrics are examples of human characteristics that have limitations. For example, there are minimum levels of contrast that our visual system can detect; humans have limits to

CHAPTER 1
Theory and General Principles

Sidebar 1-2. Human Factors Applied to Order Sets for Treatment of Congestive Heart Failure

Human factors was used to redesign order sets used for congestive heart failure (CHF). The result was significant improvements in utilization and compliance with recommended CHF clinical practice guidelines. More details on page 52.

Source: Reingold S., Kulstad E.: Impact of human factor design on the use of order sets in the treatment of congestive heart failure. *Acad Emerg Med* 14:1097–1105, Nov. 2007.

---

how much information they can hold in working memory; and the human hand can comfortably grip tools of only certain shapes and mass. Understanding these characteristics, which are based on applied research in human factors, can help you "see" the many ways in which a system's design guides or misguides the interaction between it and a human user. (We use the term *user* in this book to mean the *operator* or *worker* interacting with the system. This term is inclusive of any or all personnel who play a role in the health care setting, including, for example, clinicians, management, technicians, service personnel.)

HFE activities are rapidly increasing in health care organizations, industry, and policy- and standards-making groups. In health care organizations, HFE is taking on a more prominent role for understanding and dealing with patient safety issues[2] (as represented by Chapters 5–10). Policy groups and standards organizations are prominently featuring HFE in new guidance or even requirements regarding the development of medical devices—in the United States,[3–5] often through the U.S. Food and Drug Administration and ECRI Institute—and worldwide.[6–8]

Because HFE principles are easier to digest with demonstrations and personal interaction, a set of exercises is provided to get you started (*see* "Exercise 1. Gaining Insight," page 6; "Exercise 2. Practice Observing Human Factors Engineering Issues," page 7; and "Exercise 3. Human Factors Engineering Issues in Medication Administration," page 8).

In fact, the best way to learn HFE is to go back and forth between learning the technical details and doing hands-on or eyes-on activities. More examples of exercises can be found in Chapter 3, where the use of interactive demonstrations and small-group activities for HFE workshops is discussed.

MODELS AND THEORIES (HUMAN CAPABILITIES AND LIMITATIONS)

Within the discipline of HFE, you will find a number of areas of expertise, which can be broadly broken down into the following categories of human capabilities and limitations: physical, cognitive, and organizational. This section introduces the reader to some human factors principles in each of the three categories. It is not intended to be comprehensive but rather to provide readers with a sense of some of the representative topics in HFE. Readers interested in a particular topic are referred to the Appendix to Part I, beginning on page 71.

Exercise 1. Gaining Insight

Many people who are learning about human factors engineering describe a sudden, striking change in the way they "see" the world around them and find themselves analyzing everything for human factors issues. They experience a "brain flip." They say this occurs when they've suddenly come to the realization that design problems stare them straight in the eyes everywhere every day; whereas, before, they saw "people" problems.

Often, human factors educators will use everyday objects to help with this exercise. Think of some errors that you have either witnessed or made in your everyday routine. (You will have the opportunity to do this again in the next exercise with a health care–related activity.) This shouldn't be hard because you have likely been involved in hundreds if not hundreds of thousands of errors. For example, misreading your flight itinerary, making the wrong type of copies on a copy machine, not setting your alarm clock correctly, misprogramming a DVR, pushing rather than pulling the handle of a door, flipping the wrong light switch, mistaking the volume knob of your car stereo with that used to turn up the heat, or misinterpreting a highway sign.

Challenge
The next time you catch yourself making an error, no matter how small or seemingly insignificant, restrain yourself from dismissing it because you think you weren't paying attention, weren't being careful enough, or have cast yourself as not technologically savvy. Instead, challenge yourself to think about what aspects of the design led you to do the wrong thing.

Types of Questions to Ask
- Did the door handle look as if it should be *pushed* rather than pulled? Why?
- Were there multiple light switches for multiple light fixtures? What made you flip the one you did? (For example, was it closest to the light you wanted to control?)
- How close together are the controls in your car? Does the volume knob look and feel just like the other knobs?
- Was the highway sign too small or ambiguous? Was the sign located in the proper place?

Summary
How can the design of a system encourage error and possibly lead to an adverse event? If you begin to answer questions like those above, you will begin to identify the elements of design that influence human performance, or, conversely, human error. You have completed this exercise successfully if you find yourself thinking about the design of the things around you (human factors issues) and how they can influence the way in which you interact with them.

CHAPTER 1
Theory and General Principles

> # Exercise 2. Practice Observing Human Factors Engineering Issues
>
> Observe people at work in your health care organization. Any activity will suffice (for example, meals being prepared in the kitchen, stitches being put in, a laparoscopy procedure, an IV pump being set up, drug carts being filled in the pharmacy). Then begin asking questions like the ones listed below. Like the previous exercise, these questions will cue your thoughts toward human factors issues.
>
> ☐ How do they use their tools, paper forms, or equipment?
> ☐ Are they using shortcuts? If so, why?
> ☐ What aspects of the work area hinder their work?
> ☐ Is lighting sufficient?
> ☐ How do they arrange their tools or equipment? Why?
> ☐ What do they look at to get the job done?
> ☐ Is some information missing, hidden, or "lost in a sea" of trivial information? How do they compensate?
> ☐ Are signs, labels, and warnings legible and readable?
> ☐ How noisy is the work environment?
> ☐ How often do they get interrupted?
> ☐ How long was their shift?
>
> After completing this exercise, work through Exercise 3, which provides a scenario of an adverse event and leads you through specific questions that you can ask. At the end of that exercise, you can compare your findings to a sample list of human factors issues.

Cognitive Capabilities and Limitations

Designing a system to accommodate the cognitive capabilities and limitations of humans is crucial to optimizing the reliability and efficiency of human performance. Unlike physical ergonomics, in which you can more easily identify a mismatch between the system and physical human characteristics (mismatches are often manifested by injuries such as cumulative trauma disorders [for example, carpal tunnel syndrome or "white fingers"]), a mismatch with human cognitive characteristics is less obvious and is sometimes manifested as frustration, inefficiency, or errors.

Human Information Processing Model

The way in which humans interact with the systems in their workplace and with the environment around them is influenced by multiple factors. These factors include the design of the system and how it presents *information* to the human, characteristics of human cognition and how we *perceive* and *process* information, and how the system allows the human to manipu-

Exercise 3. Human Factors Engineering Issues in Medication Administration

Scenario: An adverse event just occurred in which the wrong medication was administered to a patient. You must determine what factors contributed to the event.

The first step is to refrain from concluding that "the person misread the label" or "he or she wasn't paying attention," or "he or she was careless." After all, if you remove that particular individual, would you be confident that others wouldn't make the same mistake ever again? The second step is to observe the process and seek answers to questions like those listed below. When you've answered these questions, you will be in a better position to identify the relevant human factors issues (*see* page 9).

- ☐ How many packages do they have to sift through?
- ☐ Where in the storage area are they looking? Why?
- ☐ How is the storage organized? Does that stay the same?
- ☐ Are there any medications put in the wrong place? Why?
- ☐ How many users retrieve medications from this storage? How often?
- ☐ What similarities exist between various packages?
- ☐ How do the packages differ in layout of information?
- ☐ Are all the packages oriented the same way (or do you have to tilt your head to read different packages)?
- ☐ How big or small is the lettering of information critical to the task? Compare this with the same attributes of less critical information.
- ☐ Is the contrast of lettering to background sufficient?
- ☐ Are there aspects of the packaging (color, graphics, warnings) that make that package look "busy"?
- ☐ What parts of the package do they look at first (the front, top, back)? Why? Is this how they search other packages?
- ☐ What are the lighting conditions?
- ☐ How often are they interrupted?
- ☐ What are the noise levels?
- ☐ Are they rushed?
- ☐ How many other tasks are they trying to do at the same time?

late or *control* it. Figure 1-1 (page 10) illustrates this human-system interaction. Within this figure is a human information processing model. A human information processing model describes the processes that occur during this human-system interaction. In general, humans receive input from a system (for example, user interface of a device or front end of an information system) through their perceptual senses, they process the information to develop some understanding of what is happening, and then they initiate some action or psychomotor sequence to manipulate the system. The system in turn processes that input and feeds changes back into the loop.

CHAPTER 1
Theory and General Principles

Sample Answer Key to Medication Administration Exercise

After asking yourself the questions in Exercise 3, you should begin to uncover some human factors design issues (listed below in no particular order). These are just a sample of the kinds of issues that a human factors engineering analysis might uncover.

1. The labeling on the medication package might be difficult to read because of small font size, low-contrast lettering, or letters or words spaced too closely.
2. There may be low light levels in the storage area, exacerbating the readability problem.
3. The package may contain too much information or distracting colors, obscuring the more critical information.
4. Critical information, such as drug name and concentration, was not displayed very prominently or was masked by other more prominent but less critical information.
5. The drug name may have been long and only the first five or so letters were read and compared with the order form. The drug name is similar to another drug's name.
6. The information on the order form may have been difficult to find or decipher because of poor layout, small font size, too many instructions, or the use of ambiguous abbreviations.
7. Other medication might have had very similar packaging, perhaps more so if the package was placed on its side, like a book on a bookshelf.
8. The medication may have been located on a higher shelf, making visual recognition more difficult and making it easy to grab the wrong one (i.e., visual contact is lost when the person reaches up for the package).
9. There may have been the expectation that a certain drug was usually located in a certain area of the drug cabinet, but the cabinet was reorganized by someone else.
10. A person retrieving medications might typically scan the bottom right of a package for drug concentration, but in this case the package was designed differently and contained some other number in the bottom right, which happened to match the drug concentration sought.
11. There may have been a change to the package design, and the person, unaware of that change, was searching for a specific "look" and found the closest one.
12. A staff shortage may have increased the tasks they are responsible for and the time pressure.
13. The person may have just worked a long and difficult shift or is sleep deprived.

Note that usually a combination of several design issues contribute to an increase in risk for error. There can be interactions among the system elements. That is, a one-design issue may be harmless, but when it is combined with a design issue with another element, it might become a dangerous accident waiting to happen or a latent failure. As you will learn in this chapter, human factors issues can be related to the physical, cognitive, or organizational incompatibility between the system and humans. All three categories have some level of representation in the list of issues above.

Figure 1-1. Human-System Interaction and Information Processing Model

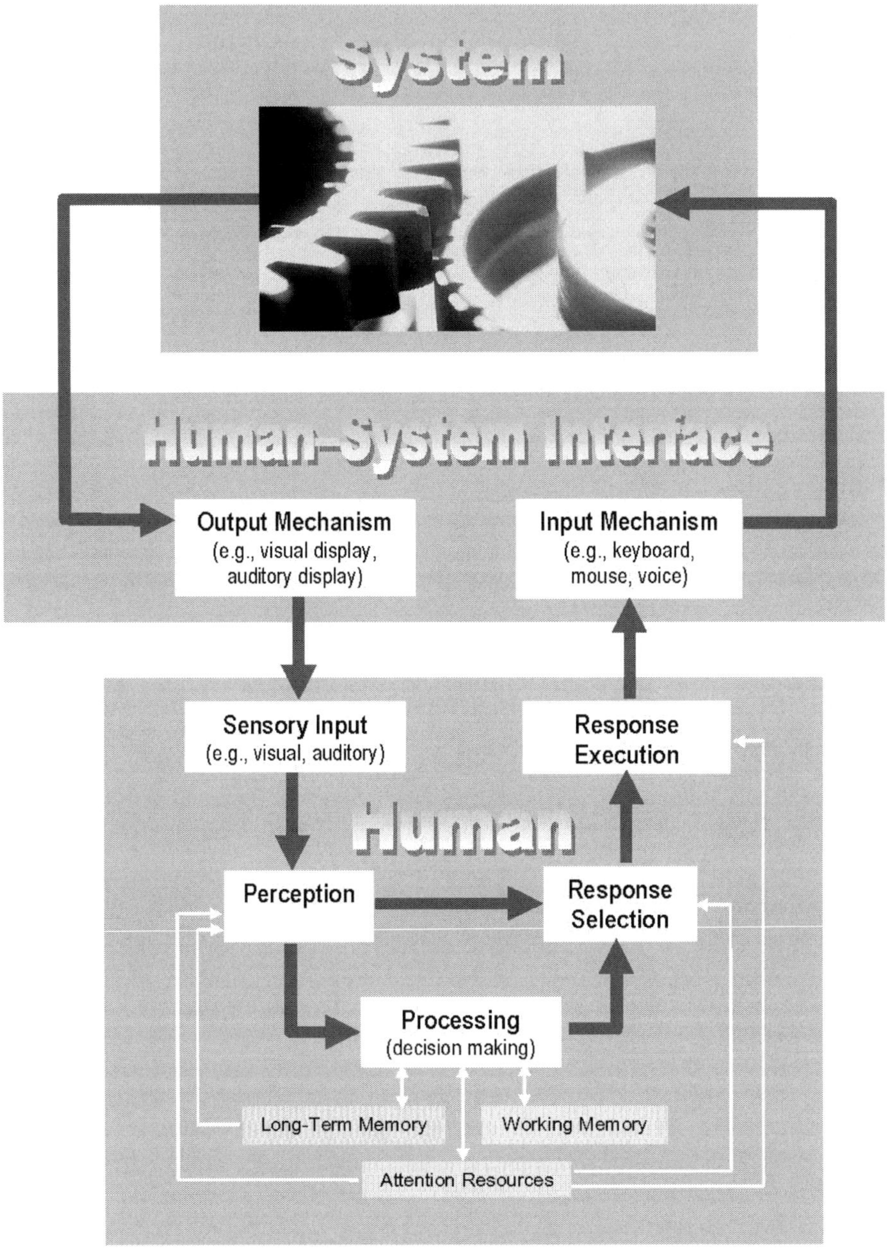

System

Human-System Interface

- **Output Mechanism** (e.g., visual display, auditory display)
- **Input Mechanism** (e.g., keyboard, mouse, voice)

Human

- Sensory Input (e.g., visual, auditory)
- Perception
- Processing (decision making)
- Response Selection
- Response Execution
- Long-Term Memory
- Working Memory
- Attention Resources

This figure illustrates the way in which humans' interaction with the systems in their workplace and with the environment around them is influenced by multiple factors.

CHAPTER 1
Theory and General Principles

Figure 1-2. Examples of Contrast

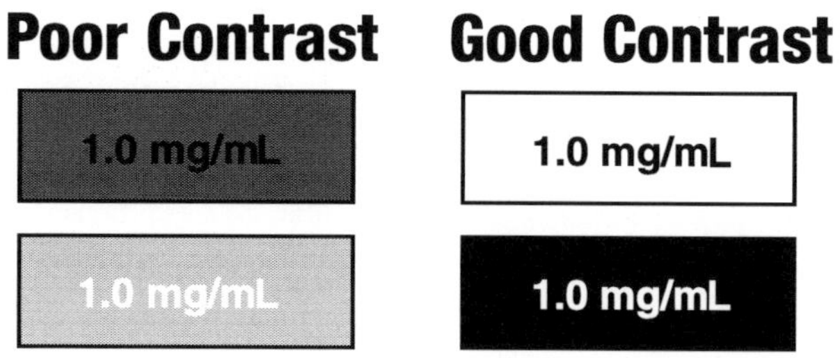

Poor Contrast

1.0 mg/mL

1.0 mg/mL

Good Contrast

1.0 mg/mL

1.0 mg/mL

A concentration of 1.0 mg/mL might be more easily confused with 10 mg/mL when contrast is poor.

Each of these stages is covered extensively in human factors textbooks. The discussion in this section provides a brief overview of three areas associated with cognition: perception, memory and attention, and decision making.

Perception

Sensory Processing Limitations

Perception is the sequence of events in which humans capture information from the world around them and process this information to develop an awareness and understanding. Human perception can process many modalities of information (stimuli): visual, auditory, haptic (touch or tactile), olfactory (smell), and taste. Other senses that provide us with information include proprioception and kinesthesis (limb position and motion) and vestibular senses. Humans have limitations in each of these modalities that restrict the detection, discrimination, or recognition of various stimuli.[9,10] We discuss some of the limitations of vision and hearing here.

Vision: Contrast Sensitivity. Contrast is the difference in luminance between a lighter area and a darker area. Luminance is the amount of light reflected off of objects in the visual field back to the eye. The ability to detect differences in contrast determines the ability to discriminate objects from each other, such as text from its background. For instance, numbers displayed on a pump might be more easily confused on a display with low-contrast lettering. An example of contrast is shown in Figure 1-2 (above).

Contrast sensitivity is the minimum difference between the luminance of a lighter area and that of a darker area that is just detectable. A reduction in contrast sensitivity occurs with the following:

- *A decrease in illumination*—that is, low contrasts are even harder to detect under low-light conditions.
- *An increase in spatial frequency* (number of light-dark pairs that occupy 1 degree of visual angle)—for example, finer print text, which has a higher spatial frequency (compared to large print)
- *Motion*—as can be observed, for example, when you try to read road signs while driving
- *An increase in age*—usually a reduction in the amount of light passing through the cornea is seen with aging.

Readability of some medication labels or equipment displays may suffer, for instance, if used in low-light conditions. Also, older patients may not be able to read the fine text used for patient instructions for some medications.

Vision: Depth and Size Perception. Humans rely on depth perception to navigate around and manipulate objects in a three-dimensional (3D) world. The ability to do so is fairly automatic; that is, we perceive and process cues in the world to give us 3D information without much thought. When these cues are absent, such as when using 2D displays in laparoscopic procedures, opportunities arise for misinterpretation of depth or location when advancing an instrument. Some of the depth cues that come into play are as follows:

- *Binocular Disparity (Stereopsis).* The lateral separation of our two eyes cause us to view objects from slightly different vantage points. The *disparity*, or slight differences between the view seen by the left eye and the view seen by the right eye, allows us to discriminate even slight differences in depth. For instance, hold two pencils at arm's length, with their tips about 10 cm apart and the sharp ends pointing toward each other, slowly bring the pointed ends together. If you try doing this with one eye closed (monocular viewing), you will find it more difficult than with both eyes open (binocular viewing). The depth cues of binocular viewing are absent when displaying information from small cameras such as in laparoscopic procedures.
- *Relative Size.* The relative size of objects can be an effective cue to judge relative depth. Size is a particularly effective cue when the viewer is familiar with the correct size of the object. However, when you are unfamiliar with the size of the object and there are no other objects in view that provide you with a sense of size, you will have trouble judging the distance. For example, if you are shown a photo of an unfamiliar object against a white background, you will have difficulty judging the size or distance the object is from the camera. However, you can judge the size and distance if you add cues of a known size to the photo such as a person holding it.
- *Textural Gradients.* Textural gradients also provide information on depth. Most surfaces have some kind of texture. When viewing a surface with texture, you will notice that the texture density (spatial frequency) increases, or becomes finer, the more distant the region. These texture gradients not only provide information to the viewer about the distance of an object, but also the slant of the surface, as well as size of objects on that surface.
- *Motion Parallax.* Occasionally, cues can be misleading as to the size and distance of objects. For instance, the Ames room (Figure 1-3, page 13) provides an illusion by distorting the structure of a room to mislead your judgment of size and distances. These illusions occur only if you stay perfectly motionless. When you move your head, you gain more depth cues. One such cue is motion parallax in which the relative motion of the objects in the field of view gives you information about their relative distance. For instance, when you look out the window of a moving train, objects that are closer to you will appear to stream past you in a direction opposite to the train, whereas more distant objects will seem to have smaller, more gradual movement in the same direction as the train.

Hearing: Range of Hearing. Humans can hear sounds that fall within a limited range of frequencies. The range of audible frequencies is determined by the minimum intensity (or amplitude), usually measured in decibels (dB), necessary to just detect a tone of a given frequency. The threshold intensity, similar to contrast sensitivity for vision, is the minimum intensity value that can be heard. The threshold

CHAPTER 1
Theory and General Principles

Figure 1-3. Ames Room

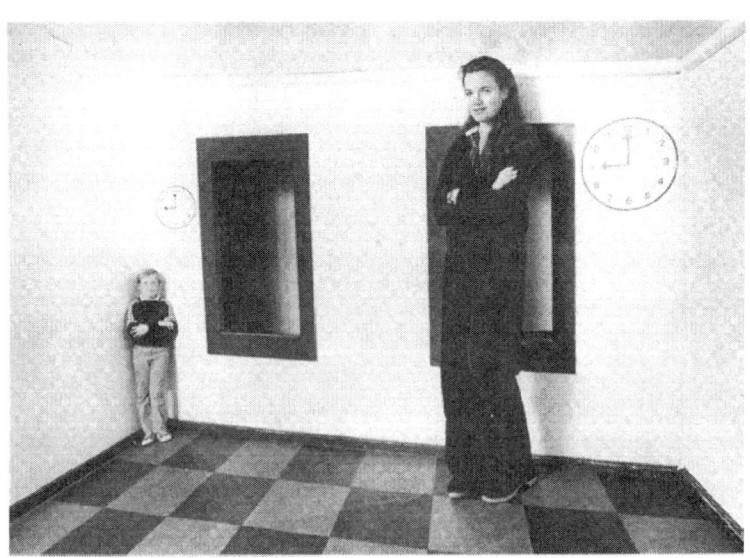

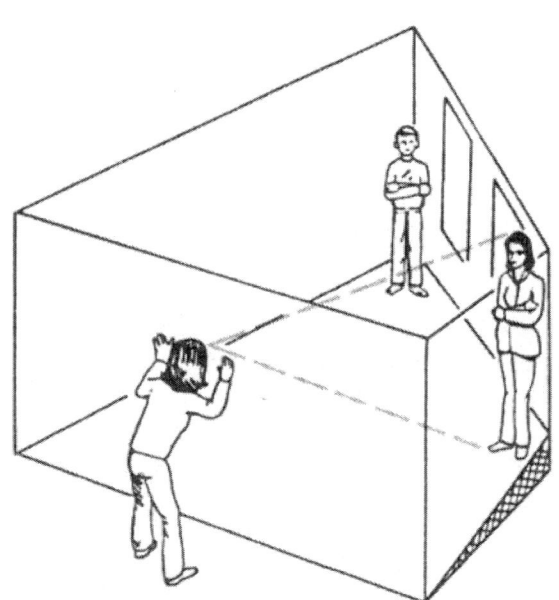

Person on the left and right are of equal size. Perceived distance influences apparent size.

Source: Sekuler R., Blake R.: *Perception*, 3rd ed. New York City: McGraw-Hill, 1994. Used with permission.

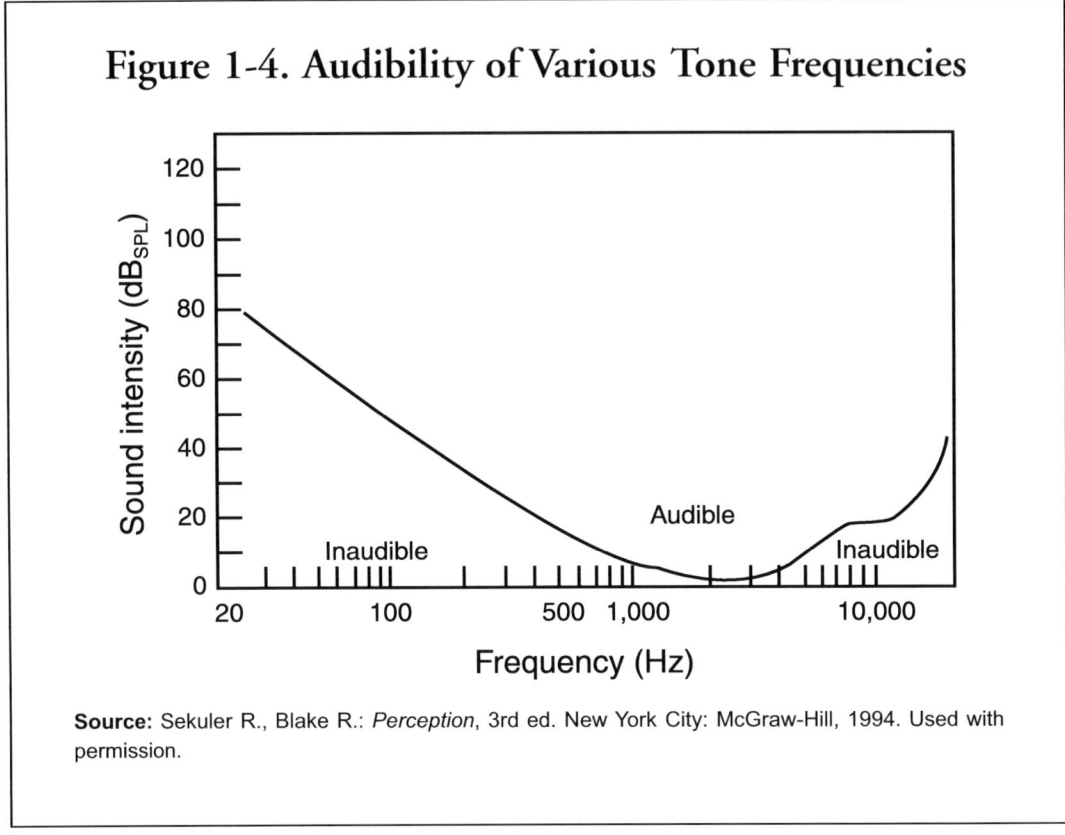

Figure 1-4. Audibility of Various Tone Frequencies

Source: Sekuler R., Blake R.: *Perception*, 3rd ed. New York City: McGraw-Hill, 1994. Used with permission.

intensity for a number of frequencies is shown in Figure 1-4 (above).

Hearing: Loudness. Loudness is the subjective impression of the intensity of sound. Because it is subjective, it is difficult to make direct measurements of loudness, although it can be linked to intensity. Perceived loudness can vary depending on the frequency (or frequencies) of the sound. To further complicate matters, loudness does not increase with intensity in the same way for all frequencies. Also loudness increases more slowly than intensity. Doubling the intensity of a sound does not double the loudness (the perception of intensity). For example, a 40 dB sound is not perceived as being twice as loud as a 20 dB sound. Also, a 10 dB increase in loudness from 20 dB to 30 dB does not sound like the same increase in loudness from 80 dB to 90 dB.

Intensity discrimination is the ability to discriminate whether one sound is louder than another. The minimum necessary change in intensity that can be perceived is called *discrimination threshold*. People typically have a discrimination threshold of about 1 to 2 dB change in intensity. When equipment alarms or auditory feedback use varying intensities to convey urgency or change in values, the change should be sufficient to allow humans to discriminate between two tones.

Hearing: Sound Localization. Our ability to localize sounds is due to the fact that we have two ears. Similar to how depth is perceived by the eyes, the spatial separation of the ears permits that information—in this case, air pressure waves from sound—to reach the ear at different times depending on the location of the sound. If the source of a sound is directly straight ahead, then the air pressure waves will reach the two ears at exactly the same time. If the source of a sound is moved to the left, then the air pressure waves will reach the left ear, the closer of the two, before reaching the right ear. This difference in time, called *interaural time difference*, provides cues that tell us where a sound is coming from.

Another cue is *interaural intensity difference*. The sound energy arriving at the closer ear will be more intense because it is located closer to the source. The occluding effect of the head, which creates a *sound shadow*, makes the sound energy arriving at the farther ear less intense. This difference in intensity provides a second cue for sound localization. The ability to localize sounds has implications for the design of operating theaters or other rooms that have several pieces of equipment (for example, the grouping of anesthesia equipment, laparoscopy equipment, operating room [OR] technician equipment) so that localization can help with identification or discrimination of alarms.

Bottom-Up and Top-Down Processing

Bottom-up processing occurs when sensory data is extracted from the world without our attention. In contrast, *top-down processing* occurs when our knowledge influences perception. For instance, knowledge controls where to place our attention (for example, *where* to search for an object), enables categorization of sensory data, guides acquisition of sensory data (*what* to look for), and supplies the context for sensory data.

Preattentive processing occurs when objects in our visual world are automatically organized. For instance, when looking at a photo, you will preattentively make the determination as to which part is the object (figure) and which parts make up the background (figure-ground perception). Sometimes, products are not designed with features that encourage preattentive processing. For example, modern medical devices often provide multiple functions or modes of operating, making it rather difficult to find the right controls for the right function. One way of encouraging preattentive processing is to spatially separate the controls for each function or to use color, shape, or size characteristics to visually group them.

Memory and Attention
Selective Attention

Selective attention is a means by which humans can filter out distractions (nonrelevant stimuli) and attend to the stimuli that are sought after. Selective attention does not guarantee perception, but is a means for achieving it. For instance, selective attention is used to visually search for a desired object, or selectively focus auditory attention on one conversation and filter out noise or other conversations. The ability to filter out irrelevant stimuli and tune to relevant ones depends on salience, expectancy, and effort.

The salience of a stimulus defines its ability to capture one's attention to signal importance. Saliency can be achieved by using stimuli that are distinct or have abrupt onsets (for example, alarms). Expectancy is a top-down (or knowledge-driven) factor that drives selective attention. Attention can be placed where we "expect" to find information, such as looking at the certain area of a monitoring display to find blood pressure reading. Finally, if the effort required to selectively focus attention is particularly high, then humans are less likely to do so. For example, a fatigued driver is less likely to look behind to check the blind spot when changing lanes.[11] We can also see many examples of this in software systems used in health care. When clinicians must dig through several levels of menus or links to find information, they are less

Divided Attention

Divided attention occurs when mental effort is allocated to two or more tasks or mental activities. *Single resource theory* states that there is a single pool of limited mental resources (or attention capacity) available to divide between tasks, and so a more demanding or difficult task will leave fewer resources available to allot to a second concurrent task. As a result, the performance of one of the tasks will suffer. For instance, most people can drive and carry on a conversation at the same time; however, if driving conditions are difficult, conversation might decrease or cease. Similarly, if the conversation becomes difficult (for example, involves problem solving), then fewer resources are available to dedicate to the task of driving, potentially compromising safety.[10,12]

Another theory, *multiple resource theory,* argues that there are multiple pools of mental resources (attention capacity), and performance declines only when two tasks share the same resources. Resources fall within categories determined by four dimensions: modality (visual versus auditory), code (spatial versus verbal), processing stage (perceptual, working memory, versus response), and visual channel (focal versus ambient). If two tasks share the same resources in one or more of these dimensions, then task interference is more likely to occur.[11,13,14] For example, speaking to someone while rehearsing a medication name will likely interfere with each other because both involve the same dimension (*verbal code*). However, less interference may be experienced if you are performing one task that involves verbal code (for example, rehearsing a medication name) while the second task involves *spatial code* (for example, tracking the trend on a patient monitoring screen).

Memory

Working memory, also sometimes called *short-term memory,* is limited in its capacity and is relatively transient; that is, we can use it to temporarily store information for short periods of time. An example of this is looking up medications listed on an order form and keeping it in your working memory until you locate it in the drug cabinet, or remembering the first part of a sentence as you listen to verbal instructions to integrate it with the second part to understand the whole sentence.

The *capacity* of working memory is limited to approximately 7 ± 2 *chunks* of information. A *chunk* is a unit of working memory space that can hold either a single item or a chunk of related items. For instance, an unrelated sequence of letters such as X P G D H is considered five chunks. However, a five-letter word such as PAPER is only one chunk, because the letters are bound together into one meaningful unit. Another limit to working memory is how long information remains in memory before it decays. Working memory *decay* is reported to be about 7 seconds for three chunks of information before recall is reduced to half and about 70 seconds for one chunk of information.[15,16]

As an example, in one strategy that is sometimes used in checking the settings of a patient-controlled analgesia (PCA) pump, nurses will remember a sequence of numbers: 2 – 5 – 6 – 30 to represent 2 mg/mL concentration, 5 mg dose, 6-minute lockout, and 30 mg per four-hour limit. They have approximately seven seconds to check this against the order form before recall of this information becomes more and more unreliable. Delays may occur if the pump is not designed to show all the settings at once—and the nurse has to scroll through several pages—or if the PCA order form is not organized in a way that allows the nurse to

CHAPTER 1
Theory and General Principles

easily find these numbers (or if the numbers appear in a different order on the form).

Whereas working memory is used to store information for immediate use, *long-term memory* allows us to store information and retrieve it later on. This is the process behind *learning*. The ability to successfully retrieve items from long term memory is influenced by a number of factors. The strength of an item influences the ease of retrieval of that item from long-term memory and is determined by (a) how frequently it is recalled and used, (b) how recently it was recalled and used, and (c) how significant it is in relation to our personal values, fears, and desires. Ease of retrieval is also influenced by associations of that item with other items. The strength of an association also depends on the frequency of recall or use.

There are several ways in which information is organized in long term memory. Information may be stored as a *cognitive map* (for example, an image of a city and its streets), which is essentially a mental representation of spatial information; a *schema*, which usually describes a sequence of activities or structured organization of knowledge on a topic; or *mental models*, which represent an understanding of how a particular system or device works and how to use it.

Decision Making

The decision-making process can be broken down into several stages: extraction of information or cues, generation and selection of a hypothesis, and generation of a plan and selection of an action. These decision-making stages depend on a number of cognitive resources, including memory and attention. Because these cognitive resources have inherent limitations, they create *biases* that affect decision making.

Biases in Decision Making

- **Cue Salience.** *Cues* that are perceptually more obvious or *salient* are more likely to gain attention and receive more weight. Sometimes, the most salient cues are not necessarily the most critical to the decision at hand. A loud equipment alarm might be irrelevant because the threshold was set too low, but it might nonetheless grab attention away from other more critical variables.
- **Cue Primacy.** When a sequence of information or cues is presented, people have the tendency to remember and attach more importance to the ones received first. In this *primacy effect*, people tend to ignore subsequent cues. This often leads to *anchoring* on an initial hypothesis (for instance, in making a diagnosis). Inability to factor in later cues is also influenced by limits on attention, as may be the case when failing to consider newly occurring back pain in a patient with abdominal aneurysm, who was first diagnosed with myocardial infarction based on chest pain and past cardiac history.
- **Cognitive Tunnel Vision and Confirmation Bias.** *Cognitive tunneling* occurs when we become anchored on a hypothesis. This anchoring is compounded by a phenomenon known as *confirmation bias*, which is the tendency to look for information that confirms a given hypothesis rather than refutes it (for example, generating an initial diagnosis and looking for the signs and symptoms that confirm it).
- **Memory Limits.** Working memory limitations constrain people to generate only a few hypotheses. People tend to consider small subsets of possible hypotheses rather than the entire relevant hypothesis due to this limitation. For instance, during a patient workup, a clinician may consider only a few diagnoses, such as myocardial infarction and pleuritis with a patient experiencing chest pain. Working memory limits (7 ± 2) can be

quickly reached when trying to factor in findings from patient history, physical exam, and test results.

Decision-Making Processes

One model of decision making is based on the *skill-, rule-, and knowledge-based* model of behavior. This model describes three kinds of decision-making processes that can be adopted, depending on the decision situation and the decision maker's level of expertise. When persons are extremely skilled at a task, the tendency is to operate at the *skill-based level* because they can generate an automatic response to the cues they perceive, without interpreting the cues, generating hypotheses, or generating plans for action. The cues automatically guide their responses, so there is minimal demand on their attentional resources. For example, highly skilled surgeons with a large repertoire of experience to draw on might be able to automatically recognize their next action based on what they "see."

When persons are less experienced at the task, then they will operate at the *rule-based level*, in which the cues are recognized as an indication of a certain state. This then triggers a set of rules which are accumulated from past experiences (for instance, following formal procedures). These rules may be either recalled from memory or retrieved from written material (as in formal procedures). Surgeons in training might use the same cues as highly experienced surgeons but they may go through a process of assessing what the current situation is to trigger a set of appropriate actions for the next step.

In novel situations, when there is no experience or rules to draw on, people operate at the *knowledge-based* level. In this type of situation, a person must integrate and understand the cues presented and identify the state of the system based on his or her knowledge to create a plan or select actions.

In another model of decision making—*recognition-primed decision making*—decision-making behavior is driven by experience such that patterns of cues are recognized by an expert, who then recalls and implements a course of action appropriate to that situation. This rapid recognition and link to an action is dependent on the availability and wealth of past experience on which to draw. Although recognition-primed decision making is similar to skill-base decision making, it explains behavior in novel situations differently. In situations in which the decision maker may not be sure of the appropriate course of action, evaluation of actions occurs by *mentally simulating* what might happen if that course of action is selected.

Design Systems to Accommodate Human Cognitive Limitations

The previous discussion illustrates how we perceive and process cues in our world to drive cognition. Knowledge of these human characteristics in cognition provides the basis for many human factors design guidelines. In designing systems that involve cognition, the system is often referred to as a *display*. A display may include the following:

- Labels on medication or IV products
- Text or numbers printed on syringes
- Preprinted order forms
- Programming interface of an IV pump
- The interface of a ventilator machine
- User interface of a computerized provider order entry system
- Incident reporting system

Essentially, anything that presents information for a human to perceive and understand can be considered a display. The principles of display design generally fall into four categories—perception, mental models, attention, and memory.

CHAPTER 1
Theory and General Principles

Examples of HFE Guidelines in Perception
Make displays legible or audible. Visual and auditory information should be presented in a way that takes into account human perceptual characteristics such as contrast sensitivity, illumination, noise, or sound intensity. For example, labels or IV pump displays should have sufficient contrast to be legible to a nurse working at night in low-light conditions.

Provide redundant cues. Displays should exploit the use of redundant cues—that is, information should be conveyed in two or more ways. Two examples would be traffic signals that use color *and* position to convey meaning (for example, red and top) and alarms that use visual *and* auditory indicators. In health care, this may have implications for designing everything from patient identification bands (for example, photo *and* name) to IV solution bags (for example, shape *and* label). A lack of redundant cues could contribute to a medical error, possibly resulting in patient harm. For example, a defibrillator/pacemaker that does not have redundant cues to indicate that it is pacing a patient may be inadvertently turned off when leads are covered by a privacy curtain.[17]

Ensure discriminability. Designers should maximize discriminating features. Symbols or words that are similar can cause confusion, either at the time they are perceived or after a person retrieves them from working memory. The extent of similarity is a ratio of similar features to different features. For instance, RTHP45 is more likely to be confused with RTHP65 than is 45 with 65 because the ratio of similar elements to different elements is greater. Designers should highlight the different elements to create better discriminability. Examples of poor discriminability in health care include similar drug names (for example, Zyrtec and Zantec)[18] and inadequately marked syringes (because there are few features to indicate how they should be used or the type of ports with which they should be used).

Examples of HFE Guidelines in Mental Models
Products or information should be presented in a way that leads the user to form a correct *mental model* of what the system is and how it operates or behaves. For example, epinephrine auto-injectors that look like pens (or use trade names invoking the mental model of a pen) but do not operate like pens are inviting user errors.[19]

Examples of HFE Guidelines in Attention
Adhere to the proximity compatibility principle. In many computerized displays, or even printed displays, information resides on multiple pages or areas of a screen. The proximity compatibility principle states that multiple sources of information that must be mentally integrated to carry out the same task should have close proximity (in the work area or on a display). The proximity can be achieved spatially (for example, locating sources of information close together) or by using color, background lines, or patterns to tie these elements together. When proximity is not achieved, it can result in confusion or errors. One example of proximity compatibility is when electronic orders for a particular patient can be accessed only at the nursing station, yet medication administration activities are completed at bedside. Without the ability to view the orders at closer proximity to these activities, nurses are required to perform mental integration of information from disparate locations.

Facilitate divided attention. In many situations, clinicians must attend to multiple pieces of information simultaneously, resulting in divided attention. For example, when using patient-monitoring equipment, clinicians must synthesize various pieces of information to determine the patient's status. To facilitate divided attention, information should be presented in a way that allows the clinician to process two or more pieces of information in parallel rather than serially. One way to do this is to present information in different modalities. For example, a patient monitor could display electrocardiograph wave forms visually, while presenting pulse information auditorily. The clinician would thereby be able to divide his or her attention between listening to the frequency and intensity of the beeping and observing the visual display.

Examples of HFE Guidelines in Memory

Minimize memory load by putting "knowledge in the world." Because of limitations in human memory, it is important to design systems so that knowledge is represented in the display to minimize users' reliance on working memory or long-term memory to retain information. An example of forcing reliance on working memory is requiring users to remember and reenter a patient name or drug name several times on multiple screens of a drug-ordering system.

Be consistent. When users become acquainted with a system, their actions may become automatic. This automatic behavior is based on a set of expectations that they develop of the system, governing the way they try to operate or interact with it, even when that behavior is no longer appropriate. When designing (or evaluating) systems, consistency with these expectations is an important factor. For example, if there are multiple information systems (such as computerized order entry, electronic charting, and an incidence reporting system) used by clinicians, there should be consistency among them. Also, organization of the information between the screens should be consistent, as in the following:
- Functionality of buttons
- Color coding (a certain color should mean the same thing) across applications
- The navigating scheme (for example, the enter key is used to move across data entry fields, or the escape [ESC] key always takes you back *one* screen)

Human-Computer Interaction (HCI) Interface Design Principles

There are also guidelines specific to designing (or evaluating) computer-based applications. When dealing with computer-based systems (which represent a significant proportion of electronic systems in health care), the interaction between the user and the computer is often termed *human-computer interaction* (HCI). The principles of HCI design are listed below.[20] Note that many overlap with the principles discussed in the previous section.

Use simple and natural dialogue. Keep the user interface as simple as possible. Additional features or functions usually add more screens or information that the user must sift through. The interface should match the user's task such that it minimizes the amount of navigation required and provides information that the user needs when it is needed and in the most useful format.

Speak the user's language. Language refers not just to verbal elements of the user interface but also to icons or other graphics. Terminology and icons should be nonambiguous and familiar to users. Also, the user interface should match the user's understanding of what is presented to him or her and how to manipulate it. Use of metaphors is one way of achieving this, such as using file folders to organize documents on a computer system.

Minimize user memory load. Humans have a much easier time recognizing than recalling information. Therefore, when options are presented from which to choose, they should be presented in parallel, such that the user can examine all options simultaneously. Populating fields automatically so that users do not have to rely on working memory is also preferred. Providing acceptable ranges for data entry (for example, enter a value: [0–20]) or the correct format (for example, enter a date: [mm/dd/yy]) is another strategy to minimize dependence on working memory.

Be consistent. Users will gain proficiency sooner and be more confident in exploring a system if there is consistency. The same information should appear in the same location on all screens and dialogue boxes, commands or functions should perform the same action in different circumstances, and terminology and symbols should be used consistently.

Provide feedback. Feedback is the information conveyed to the user about what the system is doing and the status of the user's input. Feedback should also convey to the user what actions can be performed in any given situation, and what the consequences of those actions would be. Feedback should be visible to the user, unambiguous, and meaningful.

Have clearly marked exits. Giving users clearly marked exits allows them to easily cancel or "undo" an action or escape from an undesirable situation and return to a previous screen or state. The provision of such exits will enable users to be more willing to explore a system and not feel trapped or out of control of the system.

Make shortcuts available. When users become proficient at using a system or use certain parts or functions of a system frequently, there should be shortcuts available to them. Shortcuts might include command sequences or function keys that can carry out an entire sequence of actions or placing most frequently used buttons where users use them most.

Provide meaningful error messages. When an error or fault occurs, "good error" messages will inform the user as to what happened and what he or she should do. Messages should use natural and nonintimidating language (avoid using codes or words like "fatal error" or "illegal action"), be precise about the problem rather than vague, and provide information that helps the user determine how to solve the problem.

Prevent errors. Avoid designing a system that makes it easy for a user to make an error. Some situations are more susceptible to user errors such as forcing users to spell out file names or directory paths rather than selecting from a list. Also, the use of modes can create situations in which a user can get stuck in a certain mode and not realize it or cannot get out of it. Some familiar modes include demo mode, insert mode (when you hit the insert key of a keyboard while using a word processor), or view-only/nonediting mode.

Physical Capabilities and Limitations

One of the more obvious considerations when designing systems for human use is the compatibility with physical limits of the human body such as body measurements (anthropometry), physiological limits (environmental factors such as noise, climate, and illumination), and anatomical or biomechanical constraints (limits on strength and movement). These are areas of concern for the occupational ergonomist interested in preventing workplace injuries and optimizing conditions under which humans perform work.

Beware of the average-person fallacy. Contrary to common thought, designing systems to accommodate the *average person* is not recommended. No one is average in all dimensions. For instance, if a car were designed to fit an average person (with a fixed seating distance from steering wheel, pedals, and controls), then the smaller 50% of users would not be able to reach most of the controls, the steering wheel, or pedals; and the larger 50% would not be able to comfortably fit. Only a small percentage of the population would fit. Instead, designers should design their systems to accommodate a *range* of users by using anthropometric tables of body dimensions from the 5th percentile through the 95th percentile, female and male. These tables also include adjustments for light versus heavy clothing (*see* Table 1-1, pages 23–24).

For a wide range of other design applications, there are also tables for functional reach, lifting capability, and pushing or pulling capability. For example, storage areas and narcotics cabinets should be designed so that a 5th-percentile female can reach all the shelves, otherwise you may see underutilization of shelves or reorganization of medications based on individual reach limits.

Posture and Movement

A crucial concept that affects work systems is designing for proper posture and movement. The human body must assume a posture when performing work. Designing for correct posture, however, is more than just determining chair or work surface height. Understanding correct positioning of the head, trunk, arms, hands, and visual focal point are key to designing a workspace or task that allows for proper posture and movement. When a person assumes a sitting position or carries out a physical task, a variety of muscles, ligaments and joints are involved. Whereas certain postures or movements are well suited to the human body, others create mechanical stress and cause musculoskeletal ailments (common musculoskeletal complaints include those of the back, shoulder, and wrist).

Therefore, it is important to design tools and workspaces to accommodate these limits on posture and movement. For instance, the properties of electrosurgical devices (handgrip, shape, mass, and so forth) should allow neutral positioning of the hand and wrist when held. Height and distance of surfaces for lifting and moving patients should not require bending over or outstretched arms. Storage areas should also minimize the need for bending forward or twisting.

Recently, these ergonomic issues have been studied more extensively in health care. Smith et al. looked at how the height of the monitor for laparoscopy affected performance and stress of surgeons in the OR.[21] Also, several issues related to the bed monitor and other items in the intensive care unit have been studied.[22] A large research and development effort is underway in Delft, Netherlands, to examine the many ergonomic issues, such as those concerning the use of minimally invasive surgery devices in the scrub nurse's work area.[23,24]

Sidebar 1-3 (page 25) highlights some HFE guidelines in posture and movement.

Fatigue and Sleep Deprivation
Fatigue
Fatigue is the state in which "prior physical activity and/or mental processing, in the absence of sufficient rest, results in insufficient cellular capacity or systemwide energy to maintain the original levels of activity and/or processing by using normal resources."[25(p. 469)] Fatigue may result from not only prolonged periods of doing too much, but also doing too little, and can adversely affect human performance. Both can cause problems sustaining attention. For instance, during prolonged monitoring, very small incremental changes in blood pressure may be missed by an anesthesiologist whose vigilance may be diminished by the extended time period with limited activity. Kroemer and Grandjean describe different types of fatigue, which are classified on the basis

CHAPTER 1
Theory and General Principles

Table 1-1. Anthropometric Tables for Females

Body Dimensions for Female Workers in the Age Range of 18 to 45

		Dimension (in inches except as noted)				Added Increments	
		5th	50th	95th	Standard	Light	Heavy
	Dimension Name	Percentile	Percentile	Percentile	Deviation	Clothing	Clothing
	Weight (lbs)	102.3	126.1	156.4	16.6	3.5	7.0
A	1. Vertical Reach	72.9	78.4	84.0	3.4	1.0	1.0
	2. Stature	60.0	63.8	67.8	2.4	4.0	4.0
	3. Eye Height	56.0	59.0	62.5	2.5	1.0	1.0
	4. Crotch to Floor	26.8	29.3	32.0	1.6	1.0	1.0
	5. Waist Breadth	8.4	9.4	10.9	0.8	1.0	3.0
	6. Hip Breadth	12.4	13.7	15.3	0.9	1.0	1.0
B	1. Head Width	3.3	5.7	6.1	0.2	4.0	4.0
	2. Interpupillary Distance	2.1	2.5	2.8	—	—	—
	3. Head Circumference	20.6	21.6	22.7	0.6	—	—
	4. Neck Circumference	12.2	13.3	14.4	0.7	—	—
	5. Head Length	6.8	7.3	7.7	0.3	4.5	4.5
	6. Head Height	8.0	8.6	9.4	0.5	2.5	2.5
	7. Ear to Tip of Lip Length	3.5	3.6	3.7	0.7	—	—
	8. Ear to Top of Head	4.6	5.0	5.5	0.3	2.5	2.5
	9. Ear Breadth	1.0	1.2	1.4	0.1	—	—
	Ear Length	1.8	2.0	2.3	0.2	—	—
C	1. Thumb Tip Reach	26.7	29.1	31.7	1.5	1.0	1.0
	2. Chest Circumference (Bust)	32.1	35.0	39.5	2.2	—	—
	Bust Height to Floor	43.3	46.5	50.1	2.0	1.0	1.0
	Chest Depth	8.2	9.2	10.7	0.8	1.0	3.0
	3. Waist Circumference	23.4	26.1	30.4	2.1	—	—
	Waist Height to Floor	36.7	39.4	42.5	1.8	1.0	1.0
	Waist Depth	5.8	6.6	8.0	0.7	1.0	1.0
	4. Hip Circumference	33.8	37.4	41.6	2.3	—	—
	Hip Height to Floor	29.8	32.5	35.4	1.7	1.0	1.0
	Hip Depth	7.3	8.3	9.6	0.7	1.0	2.0
	5. Upper Thigh Circumference	19.1	21.8	24.7	1.7	—	—
	Gluteal Furrow to Floor	26.1	28.6	31.3	1.6	1.0	1.0
	6. Calf Circumference	12.0	13.5	15.0	0.9	—	—
	7. Ankle Circumference	7.3	8.3	9.2	0.5	—	—
	Ankle Height	2.3	2.7	3.1	0.2	0.1	0.1
	8. Foot Length	8.7	9.5	10.2	0.4	1.5	1.5
	Foot Width	3.2	3.5	3.8	0.2	1.0	1.0
	9. Shoulder Height	48.4	51.9	55.6	2.2	1.5	1.5
	10. Forearm Circumference (flexed)	8.9	9.8	10.8	0.6	—	—
	11. Biceps Circumference (flexed)	9.1	10.4	12.1	1.0	—	—

(continued)

Table 1-1. Anthropometric Tables for Females (continued)

	Dimension Name	Dimension (in inches except as noted)				Added Increments	
		5th Percentile	50th Percentile	95th Percentile	Standard Deviation	Light Clothing	Heavy Clothing
D	1. Head to Seat Height	31.7	33.7	35.8	1.25	3.5	3.5
	2. Eye to Seat Height	27.1	29.0	31.0	1.20	1.0	1.5
	3. Shoulder Breadth	15.1	16.4	18.1	0.90	1.0	3.0
	4. Hip Breadth Sitting	13.3	15.0	17.0	1.13	1.0	3.0
E	1. Hand Length	6.7	7.2	7.9	0.4	—	1.0
	2. Hand Breadth	2.7	3.0	3.2	0.2	—	1.5
	3. Wrist Circumference	5.4	5.9	6.4	0.3	—	—
	4. Hand Circumference	6.7	7.2	7.8	0.4	—	—
	5. Hand Thickness	0.8	1.0	1.1	0.1	—	—
F	1. Knee Height	17.8	19.6	21.4	0.9	1.5	1.5
	2. Popliteal Height	15.0	16.2	17.4	0.7	1.5	1.5
	3. Buttock to Popliteal Length	17.1	18.7	20.7	1.1	0.5	1.0
	4. Buttock to Knee Length	21.0	22.6	24.4	1.0	1.0	1.5
	5. Elbow to Wrist Length	8.3	9.2	10.1	0.5	0.5	1.0
	6. Thigh Clearance	4.1	4.9	5.7	0.5	0.5	1.0
	7. Shoulder to Elbow Length	11.2	12.2	13.3	0.6	1.0	1.5
	8. Elbow Rest Height	7.4	9.0	10.6	1.0	0.5	0.5
	9. Mid-Shoulder to Seat Height	21.2	22.8	24.6	1.1	1.0	1.5

Source: Baily R.W.: *Human Performance Engineering*. Englewood Cliffs, NJ: Prentice-Hall, 1982. Used with permission.

of the cause as well as the way in which it is manifested: eye fatigue (strain of the visual system), general bodily fatigue (physical overload), mental fatigue (mental or intellectual overload), nervous fatigue (overstressing one part of the psychomotor system), chronic fatigue (accumulation over the long term), and circadian fatigue (disruption in the day-night rhythm).[26]

Sleep Deprivation

Sleep deprivation is another contributor to fatigue. Sleep deprivation can occur from repeated episodes of sleep loss (less than 7 to 9 hours of sleep for adults). Tasks that involve visual activity (such as monitoring tasks), higher level cognitive activity (such as decision making), innovation, creativity, or learning new material seem to be affected the most by sleep deprivation.[27] In health care, complex decision making or vigilance is often expected of clinicians even when they are sleep deprived.

Circadian Rhythms

Other factors that contribute to fatigue are related to circadian rhythms, such as a shift or disruption in circadian rhythms (for example, shift work or jet lag) or performing work at the low point of circadian rhythms. Circadian rhythms are natural cycles in which various bodily functions fluctuate in a 24-hour cycle. For example, body temperature dips in the early hours of the morning, rises progressively throughout the day, peaks in the late afternoon

CHAPTER 1
Theory and General Principles

Sidebar 1-3. Examples of Human Factors Guidelines for Posture and Movement

Keep joints in a neutral position. Keeping joints in a neutral position minimizes the stress placed on muscles, ligaments, and joints. Postures to avoid include bending forward for extended periods of time and twisting the trunk. At the same time, work should be kept close to the body so that limbs are not outstretched.

Avoid prolonged posture and repetitive movements. Postures and movements should be varied when possible. Prolonged postures or repeated movements can be tiring in the short term and can contribute to muscle and joint injuries in the long term.

Prevent muscular exhaustion and minimize continuous muscular effort. Muscular exhaustion should be avoided because the more that muscles become exhausted, the more rest is required to recover. Also, continuous muscular effort should be limited in duration. Maximum muscular effort can usually be maintained by most people for no more than a few seconds, while 50% muscular effort can be maintained for up to two minutes before muscular exhaustion occurs.

Take frequent breaks rather than one long one. Distributing evenly spaced breaks throughout a task or workday will help to curtail muscular fatigue. Less value is gained from rest if breaks are not taken until the end of a task or day. Breaks are particularly needed when the task is demanding. Examples of such tasks include running, frequent lifting, climbing stairs, or walking while carrying a load.

---

or evening, and then declines again. Other circadian bodily functions that show diurnal trends include heart rate, blood pressure, respiratory rate, adrenalin production, and melatonin production. As a result, humans experience sleepiness during certain times of the day-night cycle. During the early morning hours, when body temperatures reach their minimum and other functions are dampened, human performance seems to suffer the most.

When the circadian rhythm is disrupted, as is the case in crossing several time zones resulting in jet lag, a person's internal circadian rhythm is out of synchrony with the day-night cycle. When this occurs, it can take several days to adjust. Similar disruption in circadian rhythms can occur with shift work, as in the hospital setting, when people are trying to perform work at a time that is at odds with the body's circadian rhythm.

Environmental Factors

When designing a work area, environmental factors, such as illumination, noise, climate, and vibration need to be considered. There are ranges of each of these conditions within which people can tolerate and carry out work safely and comfortably. Human performance or the health of the health care worker may be adversely affected if any of these environmental factors fall outside the optimal range or levels.

Illumination

Light intensity is the amount of light falling on a work surface (expressed in lux). Appropriate light intensity is determined on the basis of the activity or task (see Table 1-2, page 26), and the

Table 1-2. Light Intensity Necessary for Activities or Tasks

Activity	Light Intensity (lux)
Navigating through hallways of a building (orientation and avoidance of obstacles)	10–200
Reading or assembling objects	200–800
Visual inspection tasks, delicate or precision work (distinguishing fine details, working with tiny objects)	1,000–10,000

Source: Adapted from Dul J., Weerdmeester B.: *Ergonomics for Beginners: A Quick Reference Guide*, 2nd ed. London: Taylor & Francis, 2001; and Kroemer K.H.E., Grandjean E.: *Fitting the Task to the Human: A Textbook of Occupational Ergonomics*, 5th ed. Philadelphia: Taylor & Francis, 1997.

---

level of detail or precision that is required in the task.

Another aspect of illumination is luminance or brightness—the amount of light reflected from objects or surfaces in the visual field back to the eyes. It is expressed in candela per m^2 (cdm^{-2}). Generally, large differences in brightness between objects or work surfaces, such as those caused by reflections and shadows, should be avoided. Insufficient light intensity or extreme variations in brightness can cause deterioration in human performance. Strategies for optimizing both light intensity and luminance include using combinations of ambient and localized lighting, screening the source of direct lighting, and using indirect lighting in ceilings.

Many activities in the health care setting, from technicians calibrating equipment to delicate procedures in the OR, can be hindered by poor lighting or glare from monitors. Work performed at the bedside, such as checking IV pump settings or reading vital signs written on bedside charts, may also be negatively affected by inadequate illumination.

Noise

Excessive noise levels in the work environment can be intrusive and disruptive to a user or cause hearing impairment. The level of annoyance or disruption depends on the loudness, frequency, and predictability of the noise, as well as the extent to which the user has control over the starting or stopping of noises. As a disruptive factor, noise can interfere with communication or cause interruptions in a person's concentration, thus increasing the chance for error. Noise levels should be kept between 30 and 80 dB. Noise levels should not drop below 30 dB; otherwise, sudden noises become obvious and cause distraction. Hearing damage can occur if the noise level exceeds on average 80 dB during the course of an eight-hour workday. Initial signs of impairment include noticeable change in ability to understand speech in a noisy environment.

In addition to keeping noise levels within an acceptable range, designers should limit the duration of continuous noise levels to which workers are exposed and follow guidelines on maximum noise levels for specific types of work

Table 1-3. Maximum Noise Levels to Avoid Annoyance/Disruptiveness During Various Activities

Activity	Maximum Noise Level dB(A)
Unskilled physical work	80
Skilled physical work	75
Precision work	70
Routine administrative work	70
Physical work with high-precision requirements	60
Simple administrative work with communication	60
Administrative work with intellectual content (drawing and design work)	55
Concentrated intellectual work (for example, working in office)	45
Concentrated intellectual work (for example, reading in library)	35

Source: Dul J., Weerdmeester B.: *Ergonomics for Beginners: A Quick Reference Guide*, 2nd ed. London: Taylor & Francis, 2001. Used with permission.

(*see* Table 1-3, above). Choose quiet machines whenever possible and enclose noisy ones. Separate noisy work from quiet work and design work areas to control levels by using ceilings and acoustic screens to absorb noise. When excessive noise cannot be avoided or abated, ear protectors should be chosen based on the pitch (frequency) of the noise to provide proper protection.

In health care, noise is a common cause of interruptions, can hinder communication during rounds or shift change, and can hinder the ability to detect or discriminate between equipment alarms. Fairbanks and Caplan describe the disruptive nature of noise in emergency medical/service vehicles.[28] When testing usability of equipment, it is crucial to include representative noise to observe the disruption or interference it causes.

Climate

Indoor climate includes four important components—air temperature, temperature radiated from hot or cold surfaces, air velocity, and relative humidity. The appropriateness of the climate depends on the nature of the work (the amount of physical exertion) and the type of clothing worn. People should be allowed to control the climate when possible. When this is not possible, air temperature should be adjusted based on the physical effort required by the task (*see* Table 1-4, page 28).

Humidity levels should be between 30% (dry air) and 70% (humid air). Radiated temperature from hot or cold surfaces (for example, a drafty window) should be minimized to within 4°C (39.2°F) of the air temperature. Air velocity (or draughts) can cause discomfort during the performance of light work when air velocity exceeds 0.1 meters/second. When extremely hot or cold climates are necessary (for example,

Table 1-4. Temperature Guidelines

Task or Activity	Temperature (°C)
Seated, thinking tasks	21 ±3
Seated, light manual tasks	19 ±3
Standing, light manual tasks	18 ±3
Standing, heavy manual tasks	17 ±3
Heavy work	16 ±3

Source: Adapted from Dul J., Weerdmeester B.: *Ergonomics for Beginners: A Quick Reference Guide*, 2nd ed. London: Taylor & Francis, 2001, and Kroemer K.H.E., Grandjean E.: *Fitting the Task to the Human: A Textbook of Occupational Ergonomics*, 5th ed. Philadelphia: Taylor & Francis, 1997.

refrigerated rooms or ovens), care should be taken to protect exposed skin, and the time spent in these rooms should be limited.

Climate can influence human performance in many ways. For instance, after an emergency medical technician moves a patient from an accident site to a helicopter, heat coupled with strenuous activity may make it difficult for him or her to turn the smooth knobs on various medical equipment because of slipperiness from perspiring hands. In freezing temperatures, cold hands or use of gloves may hinder the ability to *feel* the subtle "clicks" at discrete settings when adjusting a dial, which may be particularly problematic because the clicking cannot be *heard* over the noise at the accident scene or the helicopter noise.

Vibration

Vibration can occur as whole-body vibration (for example, originating from the work platform or seat), or hand-arm vibration (for example, from handheld powered tools). Body vibrations with frequencies less than 1 Hz can produce seasickness. Higher frequencies can lead to chest pains, difficulty breathing, impaired vision, and back pain (*see* Table 1-5, page 29).

Hand-arm vibration between 40 and 100 Hz can cause reduced dexterity of the fingers, "white fingers" (reduced blood flow to the fingers causing them to turn white and feel cold and numb, or, when duration of exposure is extended, necrosis of the fingertips), or other injuries to the muscles, joints, or bones. Frequency, acceleration, and duration of exposure determine the effects of vibration (*see* Table 1-6, page 29).

Vibration can also have an effect on the ability to carry out activities that require reading or hand-eye coordination or precision. The disruptiveness of vibration in emergency ground transport vehicles is one example. The vibration that occurs during ground or helicopter transport of a patient may cause difficulty in manipulating or operating equipment (for example, pushing buttons that are too close to each other, reading displays whose text is too small, or using a pen stylus of a handheld device with precision).

Sidebar 1-4 (pages 30–31) includes some examples of human factors guidelines on how to design systems to accommodate human physical limitations.

Table 1-5. Effects of Whole-Body Vibration

Vibration Frequency	Effect
0.2–0.7 Hz	Seasickness, nausea, vomiting
1–4 Hz	Breathing difficulty
4–10 Hz	Chest and abdominal pain, rattling of the jaws, severe discomfort, blurred vision
8–12 Hz	Backache, blurred vision
10–20 Hz	Muscular tension, headaches, eyestrain, pains in the throat, disturbance of sleep, irritation in intestines and bladder, blurred vision

Source: Adapted from Kroemer K.H.E., Grandjean E.: *Fitting the Task to the Human: A Textbook of Occupational Ergonomics*, 5th ed. Philadelphia: Taylor & Francis, 1997.

Table 1-6. Effects of Hand-Arm Vibration

Vibration Frequency	Effect
< 40 Hz	Causes degenerative symptoms in bones, joints, and tendons of the hand and arm leading to arthritis in wrist, elbow, and occasionally the shoulder.
40–300 Hz	Vibrations are dampened in the tissues and cause ill effects on blood vessels and nerves of the hand, sometimes resulting in "dead fingers."

Source: Adapted from Kroemer K.H.E., Grandjean E.: *Fitting the Task to the Human: A Textbook of Occupational Ergonomics*, 5th ed. Philadelphia: Taylor & Francis, 1997.

Organizational Context

The *organizational context* in which work is carried out is another factor that influences human performance. The organizational or management structure, job characteristics, work scheduling, virtual organizations, telework, teamwork (or group work), team training, participatory ergonomics, and safety culture are all organizational factors that affect the behavior and attitudes of workers, and hence human performance. This brief introduction to organizational structure and job/task design is intended to prod the reader into thinking about the organizational dimension when considering human performance. However, to gain an appreciation of the full range of topics and concepts, the reader is encouraged to seek out textbooks and the latest literature (Appendix, pages 71–75).

Organizational Structure

Organizations can be described along two dimensions: complexity and coupling. The

Sidebar 1-4. Examples of Human Factors Design Guidelines for Accommodating Human Physical Limitations

- Select a posture that fits the job.
- Select or design tools that suit the task and allow correct posture of the hand and wrist. The weight of a handheld tool should not exceed 2 kg if it is used with one hand.
- Chair and work height specifications depend on the task. For example, a good working height for delicate work when standing (for example, drawing) is 5–10 cm above the elbow. For manual work, a good working height is 10–15 cm below the elbow, or 15–40 cm below the elbow if the work is more heavy.
- Use a sloping work surface for reading tasks (45 degrees is appropriate for reading; no more than 15 degrees for writing and other work involving the hands).
- Allow sufficient legroom for sitting and standing workstations (for sitting, 40 cm at the knees and 100 cm at the feet; for standing work, 10 cm for the legs and 25 cm for the feet).
- Design the work area to accommodate safe lifting. The work surface should allow the lifter to keep the load close to his or her trunk and not require twisting of the trunk.
- Design the load to accommodate safe lifting. Use handgrips that allow the user to grip the load with both hands rather than with fingers. Avoid tall loads, which tend to require the user to bend his or her arms to lift the load higher (to keep it from hitting his or her legs).
- Provide a suitable level of light intensity based on the task (delicate work: 1,000–10,000 lux; reading or assembling objects: 200–800 lux; navigating through hallways and avoiding objects: 10–200 lux).
- Avoid glare or large differences in brightness between objects. Surfaces in the middle of the visual field should not have a luminance contrast greater than 3:1. Surfaces in the middle field and outer rim of the visual field should not have a luminance contrast greater than 10:1.
- Keep noise levels between 30 and 80 dB.
- Separate noisy work from quiet work.
- Use acoustic screens or ceilings to absorb noise.
- Ear protectors should be used based on the nature of the noise and the user.
- Adjust air temperature depending on the nature of the task (sedentary work: 18–24°C [64.4–75.2°F]; light manual work: 15–21°C [59–69.8°F]; heavy work: 13–19°C [55.4–66.2°F]).
- Keep humidity between 30% and 70%.
- Hot or cold radiating surfaces should be within 4°C (39.2°F) of air temperature.
- Prevent drafts (keep below 0.1 meters/second).

(continued)

> **Sidebar 1-4. Examples of Human Factors Design Guidelines for Accommodating Human Physical Limitations (continued)**
>
> - Locate tasks that are equal in physical exertion together or in the same room.
> - Limit time spent in hot or cold environments and use protective clothing.
> - Limit exposure to hand-arm vibration by alternating tasks.
> - Protect against cold and humidity when exposure to hand-arm vibration is necessary (for example, use gloves). Cold and humidity increase the risk for "white fingers."
>
> **Source:** Adapted from Dul J., Weerdmeester B.: *Ergonomics for Beginners: A Quick Reference Guide,* 2nd ed. London: Taylor & Francis, 2001; and Kroemer K.H.E., Grandjean E.: *Fitting the Task to the Human: A Textbook of Occupational Ergonomics,* 5th ed. Philadelphia: Taylor & Francis, 1997.

complexity of a system is determined by the number of subsystems that are interconnected or dependent on each other and the number of feedback loops. The *coupling* of a system is the interconnection or interaction between subsystems. A system can be tightly coupled, in which a disruption in one subsystem quickly creates a disruption in other parts of the system (such as in the just-in-time management philosophy), or loosely coupled, in which there is less disruption. In general, a highly complex system requires a decentralized management structure that empowers individual workers to make decisions and cope with unexpected events. A tightly coupled system leaves less room for error and requires a centralized management structure to carefully manage limited resources in a limited amount of time. Many cancer treatment centers, for example, could be considered tightly coupled systems, given their many interconnected subsystems. They offer a single system or location where patients visit for clinic consultations with their oncologists (medical/surgical and/or radiation), blood work, drug infusions or chemotherapy, radiation treatment, and an outpatient pharmacy. Sometimes patients go through all of these subsystems in a single day, making it expedient and efficient for the patient if the subsystems (for example, scheduling, information systems, personnel, building facilities) are running properly. Any delay or problem in any one of these subsystems would have a cascading effect.

Job or Task Design

Job or *task design* refers to the structure and components that make up a job or task. In general, a job consists of a number of tasks. Tasks can be performed by either human or machine. Some tasks are performed better by machines, whereas others are better suited for humans. In general, humans are more creative than machines in problem solving and at "filtering out noise" to focus in on specific information, whereas machines are better at counting, conducting repetitive motions, and at operating in unsafe or extreme conditions. An unsuitable task allocation is more likely to lead to dissatisfaction, injuries, or errors. Lifting of heavy equipment or patients, counting of medications (on the floors or in a pharmacy), and packing of large quantities of products are all examples of functions that may be suitable for a machine to do. Human factors analysis methods are well suited to identifying human or machine allocation because they capture task characteristics and the mental or physical demands required of the task.

The topic of job or task design itself is vast, incorporating many concepts that are both within and beyond the scope of human factors, such as employee motivation, responsibilities, autonomy, location, scheduling, team composition and division of tasks, task or job structure, and more. Human factors can be used to inform aspects of job or task design that relate to structuring of activities so that they are a suitable match to known human capabilities and limitations, thereby creating the best possible circumstances for optimal human performance and an efficient system. More in-depth study of job design can be found in the related fields of industrial engineering and organizational psychology.

CONCLUSION

HFE offers an extensive knowledge base on various human characteristics and how human performance can be positively or negatively influenced by the design of systems. In most modern health care settings, humans must interact with many systems. When systems are not designed with human characteristics in mind, the result can be inefficiency, frustration, or even errors. Recognizing that HFE is at play is the first step. However, the challenge remains to develop solutions to address the consequences of poorly designed systems. In the next chapter, we introduce various HFE tools and methods that organizations can use to meet this challenge.

References

1. International Ergonomics Association: *The Discipline of Ergonomics.* 2000. http://www.iea.cc/browse.php?contID=675 (available to members only).
2. Gawron V.J., et al.: Medical error and human factors engineering: Where are we now? *Am J Med Qual* 21:57–67, Jan.–Feb. 2006.
3. Association for the Advancement of Medical Instrumentation (AAMI): *Human Factors Engineering—Design of Medical Devices.* Arlington, VA: AAMI, 2001.
4. Harpham R., Wourms D., Pydlek D.: Understanding human factors. *Medical Device and Diagnostic Industry* 30:34–39, Feb. 2008.5
5. Pattison M., McQuaid H., Wilcox A.: Incorporating human factors in product design and development. *Med Device Technol* 18:28, 30, 32–33, Nov.–Dec. 2007.
6. International Electrotechnical Commission (IEC): *Medical Electrical Equipment–Part 1–6: General Requirements for Basic Safety and Essential Performance —Collateral Standard: Usability.* Geneva: IEC, 2010.
7. Quinn C., Stevenson E., Glenister H.: NPSA infusion device toolkit: A cost-saving way to improve patient safety. *Clinical Governance: An International Journal* 9(3):195–199, 2004.
8. International Organization for Standardization (ISO): *Medical Devices: Application of Usability Engineering to Medical Devices.* IEC 62366:2007. Geneva: ISO, 2007.
9. Sekuler R., Blake R.: *Perception,* 5th ed. New York City: McGraw-Hill, 2005.
10. Gibson J.J.: *The Perception of the Visual World.* Boston: Houghton Mifflin, 1950.
11. Wickens C.D., et al.: *An Introduction to Human Factors Engineering,* 2nd ed. Upper Saddle River, NJ: Pearson Prentice Hall, 2004.
12. Scanlon M.: Computer physician order entry and the real world: We're only humans. *Jt Comm J Qual Saf* 30:342–346, Jun. 2004.
13. Wickens C.: Multiple resources and mental workload. *Hum Factors* 50:449–455, Jun. 2008.
14. Navon D., Gopher D.: On the economy of the human processing system. *Psychol Rev* 86:214–255, May 1979.
15. Card S.K., Moran T., Newell A.: The model human processor: An engineering model of human performance. In Boff K., Kaufman L., Thomas J. (eds.): *Handbook of Perception and Human Performance,* vol 2. New York City: Wiley, 1986, pp 1–35.
16. Baddeley A.: *Working Memory, Thought, and Action.* Oxford, U.K.: Oxford University Press, 2007.
17. Gosbee J.: Who left the defibrillator on? *Jt Comm J Qual Saf* 30:282–285, May 2004.
18. Santell J.P., Cousins D.D.: Medication errors related to product names. *Jt Comm J Qual Patient Saf* 31:649–654, Nov. 2005.
19. Gosbee L.L.: Nuts! I can't figure out how to use my life-saving epinephrine auto-injector! *Jt Comm J Qual Saf* 30:220–223, Apr. 2004.

CHAPTER 1
Theory and General Principles

20. Nielsen J.: *Usability Engineering.* Boston: *AP Professional,* 1993.
21. Smith W.D., Berguer R., Nguyen N.T.: Monitor height affects surgeons' stress level and performance on minimally invasive surgery tasks. *Stud Health Technol Inform* 111:498–501, Nov. 2005.
22. Stucke S., Menzel N.N.: Ergonomic assessment of a critical care unit. *Crit Care Nurs Clin North Am* 19:155–165, Jun. 2007.
23. van Det M.J., et al.: Ergonomic assessment of neck posture in the minimally invasive surgery suite during laparoscopic cholecystectomy. *Surg Endosc* 22:2421–2427, Nov. 2008.
24. Albayrak A., et al.: A newly designed ergonomic body support for surgeons. *Surg Endosc* 21:1835–1840, Oct. 2007.
25. Job R.F.S., Dalziel J.: Defining fatigue as a condition of the organism and distinguishing it from habituation, adaptation, and boredom. In Hancock P.A., Desmond P.A. (eds): *Stress, Workload, and Fatigue.* Mahwah, NJ: Erlbaum, 2001, pp. 466–475.
26. Kroemer K.H.E., Grandjean E.: *Fitting the Task to the Human: A Textbook of Occupational Ergonomics,* 5th ed. Philadelphia: Taylor & Francis, 1997.
27. Harrison Y., Horne J.A.: The impact of sleep deprivation on decision making: A review. *J Exp Psychol Appl* 6:236–349, Sep. 2000.
28. Fairbanks R.J., Caplan S.: Poor interface design and lack of usability testing facilitate medical error. *Jt Comm J Qual Saf* 30:579–584, Oct. 2004.

CHAPTER 2
Methods and Tools

Laura Lin Gosbee, M.A.Sc.

If you've recently gained an awareness of human factors engineering (HFE) and have had a chance to walk around your health care organization taking note of all the human factors issues, you may feel overwhelmed because now you think you see a flood of human factors issues. You may not know where to even begin tackling the problems. This chapter will help you follow through to the next steps.

Consider a scenario in which you are part of a root cause analysis (RCA) team investigating an event in which a patient received an overdose of morphine while on a patient-controlled analgesia (PCA) pump. The RCA team finds that the pump was misprogrammed by a nurse, leading to an overinfusion. Armed with a little bit of human factors knowledge, you were able to persuade other RCA team members that human factors issues are to blame, but you can only come up with the same remedies that you apply to many other RCAs. As the team member responsible for carrying out the remedies, you are dreading the conversation with the nurse's manager that he should retrain his staff on how to correctly program the pump. You dread this because you know that nurses' workloads are already bursting at the seams, and they have countless other training programs already vying for priority. You also find yourself on familiar ground when you issue a memo that reminds staff to "be more careful," but you recognize that you are starting to sound like a broken record (is there a situation in which they don't need to be careful?).

Training "patches" and cautions to "be more careful" can be weak solutions if you attempt to apply them to problems that originate from HFE design issues, as can be the case in this example of misprogramming a PCA pump. The reason is that the pump may have been designed in such a way that nurses can easily enter the wrong values, such as the wrong concentration. You may prevent one particular individual from making that error again (which may have more to do with the horrifying experience rather than training), but you have not eliminated the underlying problem (in this case, a pump that has a user interface that places heavy demands on working memory, has a confusing dialogue, and uses a font that makes it difficult to distinguish between certain numbers under low-light conditions), and therefore such errors may happen again.

Even if you decide to institute special training for a larger group, your costs for putting this weak (but immediate) solution in place begins to balloon. Then you must also require training for all new employees in that wing (for as long as this pump exists), and perhaps even an organizationwide training program. Caution must be taken not to overlook the costs of extra training for nurses over the lifetime of that pump being in service in your organization, coupled with costs to defend litigation should patient harm result, heightened workload and lowered morale from equipment that is frustrating to operate, and fatigue from longer work days to fit in the new training requirements, and other costs as discussed elsewhere.[1]

To move away from this *blame and train* approach, you can adopt an HFE approach to help you devise a longer-lasting solution that tackles the problem either at the source or closer to it. Such a solution requires a bit of both art and science. Like an architect designing a building, you might infuse some creativity and innovation into the design (art), but you must also ensure that it is structurally sound (science). The science in your case is HFE, and you are ensuring a design that is sound from a human factors standpoint. As you will learn, HFE provides more than just theories and principles—it provides methods and tools to help you gain a deeper or broader understanding of the system issues. By thinking more about how design has adversely affected human performance, you should also start thinking about how you can redesign a system or modify the work environment to aid human performance. In other words, look to design and not always training. Sometimes, design can come in a form that is not readily apparent but is in the hands of the health care organization (for example, redesigning order forms or other paper forms to provide a cognitive aid to help with machine setup or operation, or changing the location of where the setup is done so that users benefit from better lighting and fewer interruptions).

SAMPLE METHODS AND TOOLS

Before looking at ways to prevent overdoses using the PCA, it is important to look at the methods and tools used in HFE analysis. HFE methods and tools fall into three general categories: analysis, design, and testing. The methods and tools may cross the boundaries of these categories because they can be used for more than one purpose. For instance, you may want to validate a new computerized provider order entry (CPOE) system that was developed inhouse. You could conduct *usability testing* to do this. However, if you are in the early or middle stages of developing this CPOE system, you can also conduct usability tests to help you *analyze* what aspects of the system's front end (user interface) cause confusion or errors, and which allows you to address them in *design* modifications.

When conducting an HFE analysis or testing of a system (for example, a design solution) to ensure its safety, the focus is placed on collecting more than just error data. Error data can give you a general idea of safeness (specifically for patients); however, the following variables also influence safety:

- *Effectiveness* (whether the system fulfills the work-related needs and functions of the clinician using it)
- *Efficiency* of use
- *Acceptance* by intended users of the system
- *Comfort* associated with the operator's use of the system

For instance, an *ineffective* system might be one that does not provide all the necessary functions to carry out a task, which results in work-arounds or circumventing steps in a protocol to accomplish a task. This mismatch in functionality can create the opportunity for error. An *inefficient* system may be one that has a long tedious sequence of steps. An overly complex or tedious sequence has more opportunity for errors than a more efficient one. A system that is *unaccepted* or disliked by its intended users may pose several problems. It may create a psychological barrier to learning correct operation of the system. Or it may be avoided and simply not used. Both create opportunity for errors. Finally, making a system comfortable for a user to operate is necessary because if it is uncomfortable to operate, chances are it defies principles of physical

CHAPTER 2
Methods and Tools

ergonomics, creating unnecessary fatigue, discomfort, or other adverse influence on human performance.

A sample of HFE methods and tools is provided in Figure 2-1 (below). The methods and tools vary in focus and depth and should be chosen on the basis of the properties of the system being analyzed or problems to be solved. For example, if you were researching the market to purchase a device and wanted a general idea of usability, you could conduct a heuristic evaluation (an audit of HFE issues) and determine if the device defies any human factors design principles that might make it prone to certain errors. However, if you have narrowed down your options and want to gain a more realistic and in-depth appreciation of usability issues associated with the candidate devices, you may want to conduct user testing, using a representative group of end users (the people who will eventually be using the devices), realistic scenarios, or tasks; and/or even in a simulated environment complete with noise, low lighting, multiple tasks, or interruptions.

Recently, a consortium of universities and industry partners in the United Kingdom started looking into the relative effectiveness of HFE methods. The Multidisciplinary Assessment of Technology Centre for Health Care (MATCH) is evaluating and translating ergonomics (HFE) methods for selection and use in a variety of projects. In an initial review of HFE methods, including usability testing, contextual inquiry, and heuristic evaluation,

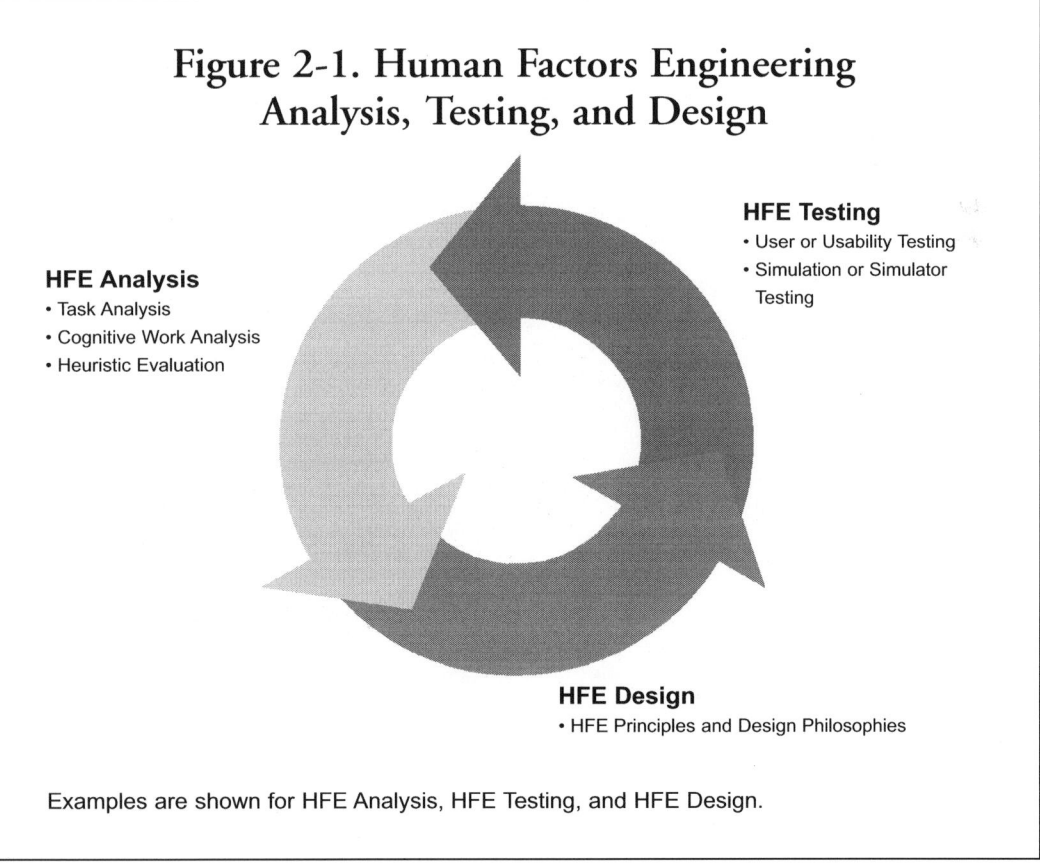

Figure 2-1. Human Factors Engineering Analysis, Testing, and Design

HFE Analysis
- Task Analysis
- Cognitive Work Analysis
- Heuristic Evaluation

HFE Testing
- User or Usability Testing
- Simulation or Simulator Testing

HFE Design
- HFE Principles and Design Philosophies

Examples are shown for HFE Analysis, HFE Testing, and HFE Design.

Martin et al. found that much remains to be learned about their optimal selection and use in health care.[2]

HFE Design

When developing a solution to HFE issues, you will need to generate design requirements on the basis of an understanding of the user population, the task, and the environment of use. Whether you are working on the development of an information system, devising a solution to storage problems, improving work scheduling, improving preprinted order forms, or planning the renovation or construction of a wing in your facility, HFE provides design guidance for physical, cognitive, and organizational aspects of your design/development project. Some recommendations for each of these areas were provided in Chapter 1, and the Appendix (pages 71–75) provides references to a variety of sources where the reader can obtain more comprehensive coverage of design principles, as well as design guidance pertaining to health care applications. A detailed set of standards about HFE design can be found in a newly approved document from the Association for Advancement of Medical Instrumentation and American National Standards Institute.[3]

HFE also provides a number of approaches or design philosophies that can help guide your development and design projects. These include *user-centered design* and an *iterative design approach*. Both are applicable to projects involving development of solutions to existing problems or development of new products or systems (discussed in more detail later).

In user-centered design, user needs, which are identified through HFE analysis methods (as shown in Figure 2-1), and human characteristics, such as those described in Chapter 1, are used to develop the design's functional and format requirements. The user-centered design approach factors in the human or user during design/development to achieve appropriate functionality and good usability.[4]

An iterative design approach is similar in that user needs and performance are of great importance. User testing is conducted at the early stages of design and conducted throughout product development to help guide and validate design modifications. By repeating this process over and over (design iterations), the final design will more closely reflect user's functional needs and there will be fewer surprises or usability problems discovered at the end, when the cost of changing or modifying will be much greater.

HFE Analysis

You can find compendiums of many HFE analysis methods, but the following offers an overview of some widely used analysis methods. When analyzing or testing a system, the methods described here can be used to focus on detailed aspects of design or on a broad swath of design issues (Figure 2-2, page 39). For example, detailed aspects of design might include the buttons or labels of a pump, the font or background color of computerized order entry screens, or the method of navigating through those screens. A broader focus may include how training on the operation of one piece of equipment might negatively influence learning on another, how noise in the environment masks the auditory feedback of the device, or whether an information system provides functions to support collaboration or information sharing with other team members.

Task Analysis

Task analysis is a tool used by HFE professionals to develop a deeper understanding of users and tasks in the context of goals to be met. It can vary in level of detail or scope, but, generally, a task analysis will consist of gathering the

CHAPTER 2
Methods and Tools

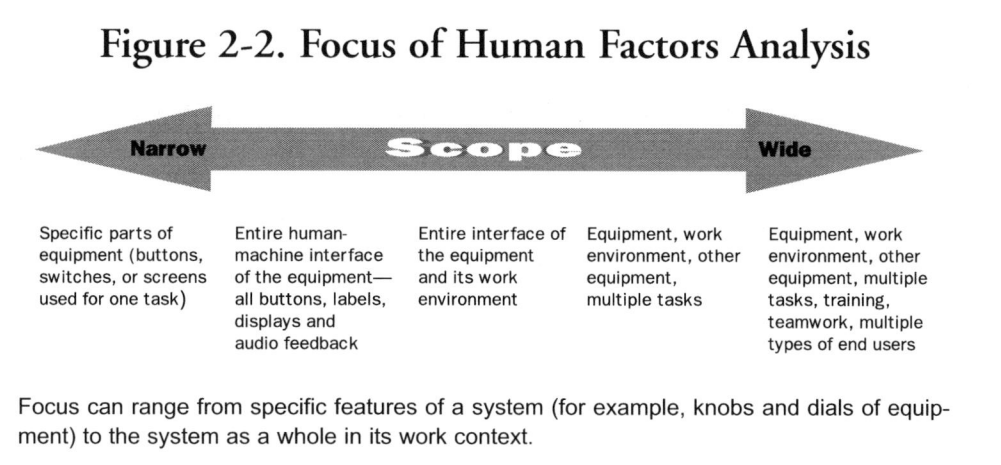

Figure 2-2. Focus of Human Factors Analysis

following data:
- Nature of the task being performed
- Activities that make up the task
- Environment in which the task is performed
- Equipment or tools used in the task
- Information required by the user to carry out the task.

These data can be gathered by a variety of methods, including observations in the field where work is performed, "think aloud" verbal protocols in which users think out loud as they perform or imagine performing a task, interviews with users, and surveys or questionnaires. Miletello applied one form of the method, cognitive task analysis, to elicit knowledge from neonatal intensive care unit (NICU) nurses on assessment of infants at risk for necrotizing enterocolitis.[5] These problem-solving strategies could potentially be used for developing nurse instruction or decision support systems. In another example, Shachak et al. used task analysis to help determine the optimal redesign of a computerized order entry system for primary care physicians.[6] Another group performed a task analysis of laparoscopic surgery to develop a procedural checklist to guide complex decisions and actions during surgery.[7]

Cognitive Work Analysis

Cognitive work analysis is a framework for analyzing complex sociotechnical systems (that is, systems, such as a hospital, "composed of technical, physiological, and social elements"[8(p. 9)]). The framework consists of five phases of analysis that examine the constraints imposed by the system and work environment that shape human behavior. These five phases of analysis focus on the following aspects of the system:
- Work domain (the behavior of the system independent of a human worker)
- Control tasks (the goals that need to be achieved, independent of who does it and how they do it)
- Strategies (how to achieve the goals)
- Social organization and cooperation (relationships between users or stakeholders and the system)
- Competencies (the knowledge, rules, or skills needed)

Sharp and Helmicki used this method of analysis to design displays that help clinicians assess neonatal oxygenation in the NICU.[9] Also, Hajdukiewicz et al. applied the method of analysis for mapping medical roles, responsibilities, sensors, and controls in the context of patient monitoring in the operating room.[10]

They also provide suggestions for medical informatics designers seeking to design novel training programs and human-computer displays.

Heuristic Evaluation

Heuristic evaluation, "systematic inspection of the user interface design for usability,"[11(p. 155)] can be used in an iterative design approach to help uncover usability issues so that they can be resolved in the next iteration of a new product or solution development. It can also be used to analyze prospective systems (for example, for procurement) or existing ones (for example, RCA) to help explain why errors might be occurring. In a heuristic evaluation, an HFE professional systematically looks at all aspects of the system and identifies aspects of its design that do not adhere to human factors design principles, as briefly described in Chapter 1. Lin et al., for example, conducted a heuristic evaluation within the context of a more extensive task analysis of PCA pumps. Redesigning the specific user interface on the basis of human factors techniques and principles led to significantly faster, easier, and more reliable performance.[12]

The heuristic evaluation technique has become a popular HFE method in health care safety research during the past 10 years, which reflects in part the relative simplicity and low cost of applying this method. There is no need to recruit participants, purchase testing equipment (other than what is being evaluated), or secure special laboratory space to conduct a heuristic evaluation. It has been applied to clinical information systems,[13] patient online education systems,[14] and pacemaker programming machines.[15] Graham et al. applied heuristic evaluation to infusion pumps to help guide improvement efforts in their critical care areas. Using four raters, they found 231 violations across a list of 14 usability design guidelines, such as "memory load is minimized" and "match between the system and the world" (adapted from computer software sets). Locating most of these design problems at the pump-loading and dose-changing steps allowed them to proactively address those areas in their in-service training curricula. According to the authors, the results could be useful for manufacturers in designing future infusion pump systems.[16]

Heuristic evaluation can also guide software development. For example, Tang et al. sought to improve the HFE design aspects of a home-grown computerized ambulance communication system. The system connected trauma specialists to ambulance personnel in real time and allowed remote access to patient data. In the first application of heuristic evaluation, Tang and colleagues found several violations in the user interface design, such as lack of feedback of system status (to confirm saving of file) and inconsistent location of key data elements (patient name in small font at bottom of screen). After the software was redesigned, the team found that the new system had fewer than half the violations.[17]

Contextual Inquiry

In contextual inquiry, a collection of tools is used to develop a deeper understanding of who the users are and the context in which they perform their tasks. In such an analysis, the work context is described using different models[18,19]:

- Flow model (how work is divided up and coordinated across people)
- Sequence model (the sequence of tasks)
- Artifact model (the objects that people create, use, or modify)
- Cultural model (expectations, values, policies)
- Physical model (the environmental factors that enable or constrain the work)

For instance, Brown applied contextual inquiry to an ultrasound system to improve its usability.[20] Also, Coble et al. used contextual inquiry to determine users' needs in designing a comprehensive clinical information system.[21] In both cases, the researchers observed clinicians using the systems in a real context and probed deeper to determine if and when problems arose. The observations and questioning allowed a deeper understanding of the work flow, task sequence, task setting, and any tools or aids that people create to facilitate their work.

Other researchers, such as Blechner et al., have used contextual inquiry (or, as they call it, contextual *design*) to examine the process by which medical students learn in various settings. Their work resulted in many design changes for the learning process and tools.[22] An example of the output of this technique is found in Figure 2-3 (page 42).

HFE Testing and Usability Testing

Usability testing is conducted to evaluate the design of a system.[23] This HFE method is considered the gold standard in finding and characterizing design flaws.[3] A usability test involves end users who perform predetermined tasks while performance metrics are gathered. The goal is always to find and improve deficiencies in the system——not the end user (*end users* are the people who will be using the device, software, or other systems). Performance metrics can include the following:
- Percentage of tasks completed
- Number of commands or features used
- Time to complete a task
- Number of errors
- Time spent on errors
- Time to learn
- Number of times help or documentation is consulted

The scope and focus of usability tests, along with the level of fidelity of the prototype and setting, can vary widely, The scope can range from a single control switch to a complex work station that fills half a room. For computer systems in development, for example, a low-fidelity paper prototype can be used to elicit the manner in which a person tries to enter data, click on "buttons," and other actions. A high-fidelity prototype would be a fully working computer system with all the screens, realistic transitions between screens, and other operating characteristics. A low-fidelity setting could be a conference room with a few props, all the way up to a higher-fidelity setting such as an ICU in a health care simulation center. More will be said about the relationship between usability testing and simulation in the next section.

Many people may think that usability testing is just another way of getting the kind of information that might be obtained in a focus group or interview. Yet it should be understood that the goal in usability testing is for the participant to get the task done in any manner that he or she sees fit. The goal is not for the participant to play around with the device and then give an opinion. In many cases, a participant's subjective preference will diverge from his or her actual performance when using the device or system, as shown by Garmer, Ylvén, and Karlsson, who compared focus group–based and usability testing–based testing.[24]

McLaughlin applied usability testing to the design and validation of crash cart medication drawers,[25] and Lin, Vicente, and Doyle 2001 conducted usability tests of PCA pumps.[26] Both of these applications are discussed more fully later in this chapter.

In addition to evaluating or designing systems, user testing can be conducted to guide the

Figure 2-3. Flow Model of Medical Student Learning Activities

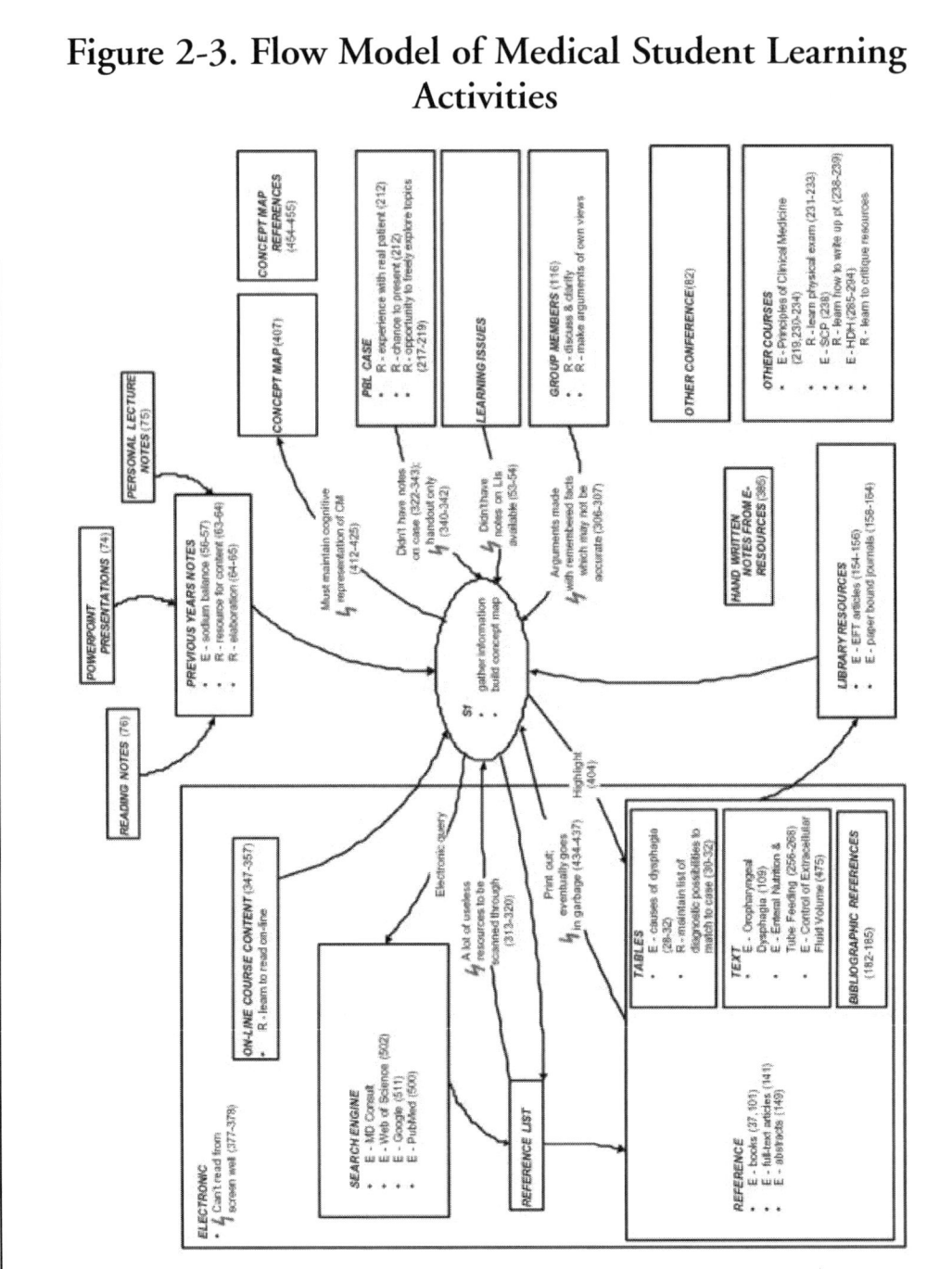

The flow model documents the communication and coordination involved in the work. Individuals and well-defined groups are represented by circles.

Source: Blechner M., et al.: Using contextual design to identify potential innovations for problem based learning. *AMIA Annu Symp Proc.* 2003. http://www.ncbi.nlm.nih.gov/pmc/articles/PMC1479946/ (accessed May 13, 2010). Used with permission.

development of training materials or implementation strategies so that they address usability issues. As an added benefit, frontline staff's participation in those tests can help promote awareness of HFE issues (*see* Chapter 6).

Merry and colleagues used usability testing to design a new drug-delivery system, which, when used by 10 anesthesiologists in mock surgical cases, resulted in statistically significant (p < .001) mean reductions in medication administration–related preoperative time (from 346 seconds to 105 seconds) and interoperative time (104 seconds to 20 seconds).[27]

Usability testing can be deployed to help make purchasing decisions among candidate devices with a relatively high cost and/or frequency of use, where failure could result in patient harm. For example, Uzawa, Yamada, and Suzukawa developed several usability test scenarios to obtain comparative error rates and times on task for four ventilator brands. As shown in Figure 2-4 (page 44), the brands' respective completion and operational failure rates for three main tasks did not suggest that any single ventilator had an advantage across all three tasks.[28]

Similarly, a study reported by Vignaux, Tassaux, and Jolliet, in which 10 anesthesiologists conducted several typical ventilator tasks in a simulated intensive care setting, showed that a mean of 13 failures occurred for all ventilator types, with no single ventilator clearly better than the others on all the scenarios.[29]

Comparative usability testing is also often conducted to guide procurement of devices, such as glucometers and inhalers, that are crucial to managing chronic disease in large populations. For example, Diggory et al., comparing performance between two brands of dry-powder inhalers for delivery of zanamivir, found that with one brand, immediately after training, 34 of 35 patients were able to correctly load and prime the device, whereas only 19 of 38 patients could do so for the other brand. Twenty-four hours after training, the devices were successfully used by 2 of 35 patients and 13 of 37 patients, respectively, which also suggested a trainability issue, which is sensitive to the most troublesome areas of design.[30]

Relationship Between Usability Testing and Health Care Simulation

Health care simulation centers include high-fidelity mock-up rooms that are mainly used to teach or assess the health care provider. For usability testing, these same resources can be used to assess devices, software, and even room layout.[31] The more realistic setting often allows an analysis of many variables in the work context that influence human performance, and they cannot easily be removed from the testing regimen without affecting the ability to generalize the results. This is particularly true for tasks that are time-critical, involve coordination among team members, and entail complex decisions with a great deal of uncertainty.

In Situ Simulation

Performing in situ simulation in frontline settings is used for both training purposes and to find systems problems that are difficult to detect by other means.[32] The manikin and simulation personnel are brought into unused rooms or units, and personnel who work in these settings are asked to go through crisis scenarios to practice infrequent events. Simulation and other hospital personnel have found the experience just as enlightening about the shortcomings of tools, workspaces, computer systems, and other accessories as discovering communication and teamwork issues. In a way, in situ simulation is usability testing done in the "field."[33]

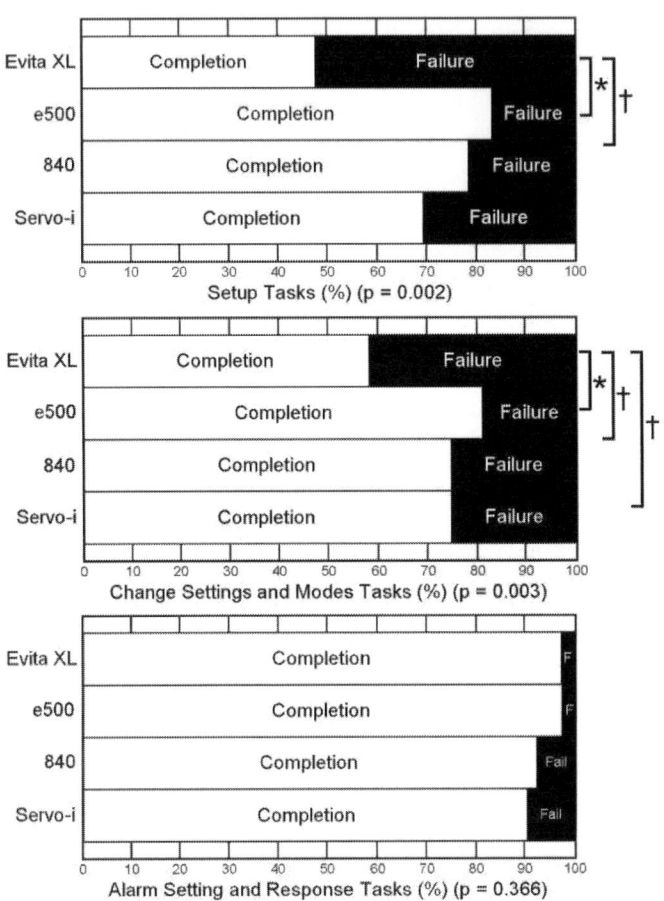

Figure 2-4. Comparison of the Number of Completions and Operational Failures Among Four Ventilators in Three Task Categories

The completion and operational failure rates of the four ventilators for setup, change settings and mode, and alarm management are shown.

Source: Uzawa Y., Yamada Y., Suzukawa M.: Evaluation of the user interface simplicity in the modern generation of mechanical ventilators. *Respir Care* 53:329–337, Mar. 2008. Used with permission.

APPLYING HFE METHODS AND TECHNIQUES TO HEALTH CARE

HFE brings forth a set of tools that are directly applicable to patient safety. In this section, we focus on four areas that can benefit from HFE tools and principles: product procurement, RCA, proactive risk assessment (Failure Mode and Effects Analysis [FMEA]), and teaching HFE in your health care organization.

Product Procurement

Any of the HFE analyses or HFE testing methods discussed in the previous section can be used to identify usability issues related to products being considered for procurement. Some device manufacturers are beginning to incorporate human factors into their product development process. Whether they have a program or not, here is what you can do:

- Ask for usability data from the manufacturer, even if you are unsure if it has a human factors program. If the manufacturer does not understand what "usability data" means, you will know that human factors is not in its vocabulary yet and it may not value usability in its products.
- If no usability data are available and you cannot get access to the product (either from the manufacturer or elsewhere) to conduct your own HFE analysis or usability test, ask for a copy of the user manual and conduct a task analysis using information presented there. It may even be possible, and highly recommended, to produce paper prototypes on the basis of the illustrations in the manual to conduct low-fidelity usability tests.
- Ask for names of other customers who have purchased the system and visit their health care facility to observe the product being used. You can conduct an HFE analysis using the information gathered from this field visit.

Note that usability data are *not* what the manufacturer says other customers have said. In fact, perceived performance and personal preference are not often consistent with actual human/user performance.

A product that has a poor user interface or is not intuitive can create not only frustration but also inefficiencies and delays—and add costs from extra training or time spent dealing with service representatives. These consequences should be factored into the costs when comparing prospective products.[1]

RCA and FMEA

When conducting an RCA—an investigation of an adverse event (or close call)—the RCA team collects a great deal of information to understand what happened and the circumstances under which it occurred for the purpose of identifying the *root cause(s)* of the event. Whereas an RCA is conducted retrospectively following an adverse event, an FMEA is usually done prospectively, as a proactive measure. As is the case with an RCA, there is a great deal of information gathering to identify the possible things that can go wrong with a system, as well as their causes or *failure mode causes*.

Root causes and *failure mode causes* generally mean the same thing. HFE analysis methods described earlier in this chapter provide systematic ways of gathering such data that cover all the bases (the human, the equipment, the work environment, and the organizational factors, and the interaction amongst them). The HFE issues or design problems identified in such analyses (for example, equipment with poorly labeled controls, work environment with poor lighting) are root causes in the RCA and failure mode causes in the FMEA.

**HFE Issue = Design Problem =
Root Cause = Failure Mode Cause**

After you have conducted the analysis portion of an RCA and have identified a root cause (or HFE issue), you generate actions or solutions. These solutions should be, as much as possible, *design solutions*—solutions that eliminate or mitigate the source of the problem. In extreme cases this might mean getting rid of an error-prone piece of equipment. Other times, it may mean redesigning or modifying the equipment, the work environment, or the task/job, so that the risk is eliminated. This could be a matter of reconfiguring equipment or software (or asking the vendor to do so), redesigning labels printed in the pharmacy, reorganizing a work area, or changing the sequence of activities for a particular task.

Whatever the design solution, you can also use HFE testing methods to test your solution before fielding it. Your solution is essentially a product that happens to be developed "in-house." As such, you should treat it as you would a procurement decision and subject it to usability testing to ensure that you are not substituting one set of problems for another equally dangerous set. An example of this process of testing design solutions is in the Code Cart example (pages 49–52).

To summarize, when conducting an RCA or FMEA, do the following:
- Conduct HFE analyses to identify HFE issues (root causes or failure mode causes). Refer to the section on HFE analysis methods (beginning on page 38).
- Develop design solutions that target the HFE issues (look to design, not training). Refer to cost-justification resources in the Appendix.
- Conduct HFE testing to ensure that your solution works, modifying if necessary. Hire an outside HFE consultant if in-house HFE expertise is unavailable.

Teaching

Usability testing and simulator testing can serve multiple purposes, one of which is as a teaching tool to convey human factors concepts. This is the case at Sunnybrook Health Sciences Centre, in Toronto, where, following a Grand Rounds lecture on HFE,[34] a follow-up lecture allowed medical students to conduct usability tests of an epinephrine auto-injector as a hands-on exercise.

In this exercise, students worked in groups of four, with one serving as the test director (Sidebar 2-1, page 47), one acting as an anaphylactic "patient" to create context, and the two students serving as the end users who had to quickly administer epinephrine (using a dummy auto-injector with no needles and no medication) to the patient experiencing an anaphylactic reaction. The "patients" acted out symptoms such as difficulty in breathing (and in one case even loss of consciousness) to convey a sense of urgency that is usually associated with use of this device in the real world. In the end, students were able to identify major usability flaws with the epinephrine auto-injector that hindered correct operation of this life-saving device. Most of the students reported that the exercise gave them an awareness of human factors issues and an appreciation of how design affects performance, which was the broader goal of the exercise.

In summary, HFE training can be offered to frontline clinicians, risk managers, shift managers, residents, or students (medical, nursing, pharmacy, biomedical) so that they can help identify HFE problems throughout the health care organization. This training can be augmented by providing opportunities to conduct or observe usability testing or participate in simulator testing or simulator training.

EXAMPLES FROM THE LITERATURE
PCA Pumps
At the University of Toronto, HFE researchers began investigating PCA pumps after hearing nurse complaints at an affiliated teaching hospital (Toronto General Hospital [now University Health Network]) about a recently purchased pump. Although the information was anecdotal, there was reason to believe that design issues were at play, which led to a human factors study of the pump.[12,26]

Analysis
The first phase of the study involved a human

CHAPTER 2
Methods and Tools

Sidebar 2-1. Test Director's Script Used by Medical Students to Conduct Usability Testing

Protocol and Director Script:
☐ Start the test by getting the first participant from outside
☐ Read this script to him or her:

> "We are evaluating a device today and want to see how easy or difficult it is to use. This device does not have any needles or medication, so you can't get hurt or hurt anyone."

> "We have a patient here with severe peanut allergy. He/she is having an anaphylactic reaction. You need to administer this epinephrine auto-injector quickly!"

☐ Give the epinephrine auto-injector to the participant. Note the start time: _____
☐ Observe, and don't help.
☐ Note how the participant tries to use it (correctly or incorrectly). Note what he or she struggles with. Note whether the following steps are performed correctly:

  ☐ Takes grey cap off.
  ☐ Puts black tip against thigh.
  ☐ Uses jabbing motion to activate the epinephrine auto-injector.
  ☐ Holds in place for 10 seconds.

☐ Stop the test once your participant "thinks" he or she has administered it correctly. Note the stop time: _____
☐ Explain to the participant how to correctly use it. And say that the first participant can observe the second participant (no helping).
☐ Get the second participant from outside and repeat test.

---

factors analysis of the pump. HFE researchers conducted a cognitive task analysis and a heuristic evaluation, two of the analysis methods described earlier in the chapter. Data were gathered using field observations, bench tests, questionnaires, and the pump's user's manual. The heuristic evaluation helped the HFE professionals identify which design principles were violated and hence which aspects of the pump's design could lead to programming errors.

Design
The second phase involved redesigning the PCA pump's programming interface on the basis of the results of the cognitive task analysis and heuristic evaluation. The redesigned PCA pump included such features as logical grouping and labeling of controls, simplified and more natural language in the displayed messages, and improved status display and feedback (Figure 2-5, page 48). The redesigned interface was accompanied by a redesign of the programming sequence (Figure 2-6, page 49).

Testing
In the third and final phase, a computer simulation of the redesigned pump's programming interface was empirically evaluated with users.

Figure 2-5. Patient-Controlled Analgesia Pump Programming Interface

a. Existing Design

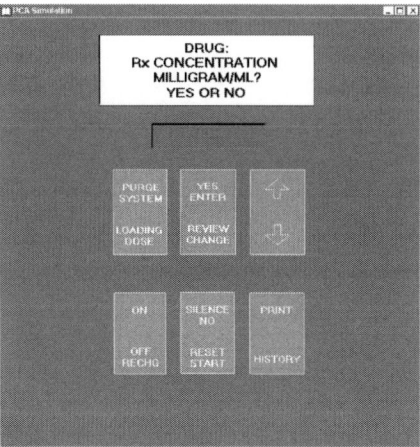

b. New Design

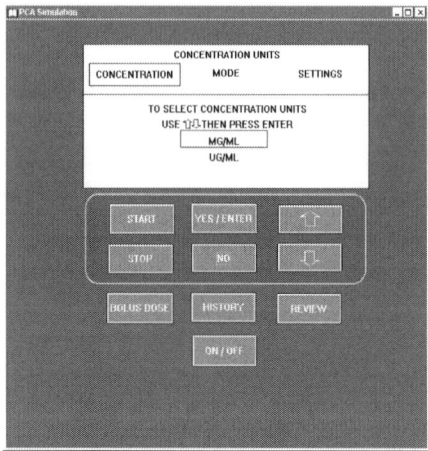

The figure shows the existing (a) and (b) redesigned interfaces.

Source: Lin L., Vicente K.J., Doyle D.J.: Patient safety, potential adverse drug events, and medical device design: A human factors engineering approach. *J Biomed Inform* 34:274–284, Aug. 2001. Used with permission.

The testing involved two user groups: novice users (nursing students with no previous experience with pumps) and experienced PCA users (recovery room nurses). After some training and practice, participants were given a PCA order form (prescription) and were asked to program the pumps using each interface. Performance data were collected, including time to complete each programming task, number of errors, and subjective workload (for example, mental effort, frustration).

Both user groups showed marked improvements with the redesigned PCA pump. There was a 50% reduction in errors for nursing students and a 55% reduction in errors for nurses. There were no errors in setting the drug concentration with the redesigned pump, demonstrating a degree of resistance to the most culpable error found in the medical device reports.[10,12]

Improvements were also shown in task completion time. The nurses showed 18% faster completion times despite having no previous experience with the new system, compared to several years of experience with the existing pump. This improvement can be attributed to, among other things, the fact that significantly fewer programming errors were made, and thus less time was wasted recovering from errors. Both user groups also reported lower levels of subjective workload with the redesigned interface compared to the existing pump: 53% and 14% lower for nursing students and nurses, respectively. Also, postexperiment interviews

CHAPTER 2
Methods and Tools

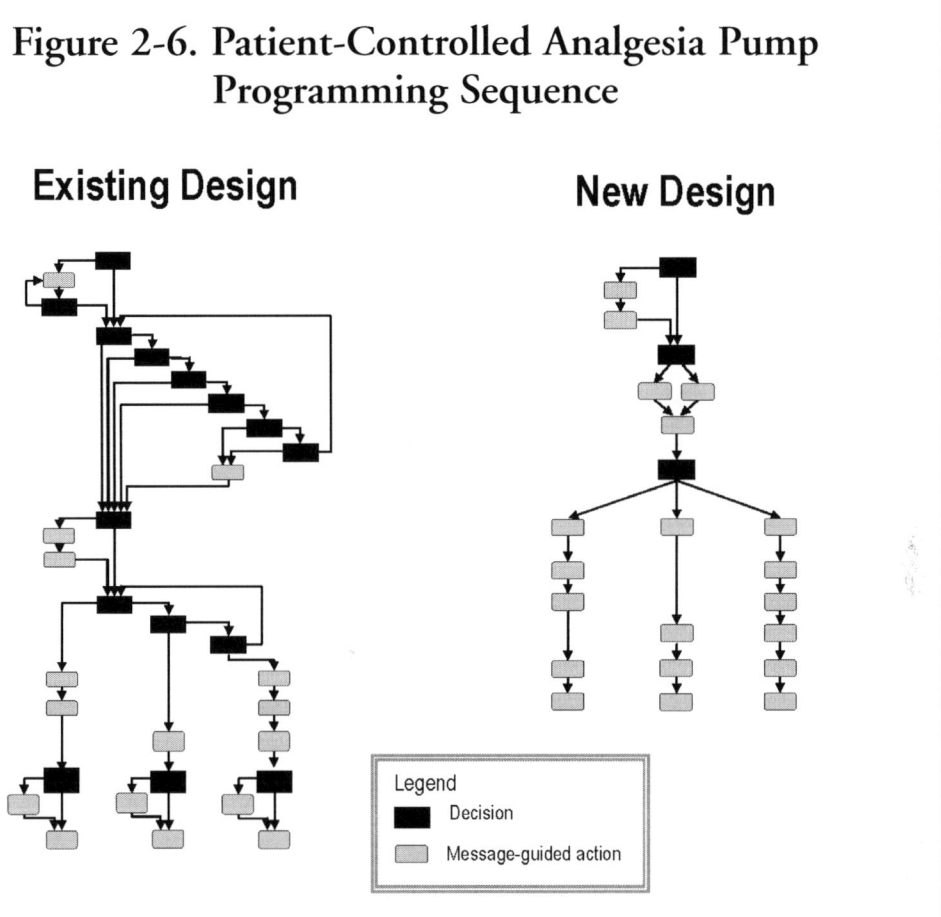

Figure 2-6. Patient-Controlled Analgesia Pump Programming Sequence

As the figure shows, the complexity of the programming sequence (a) was reduced in the redesigned interface (b) such that programming could be accomplished with fewer steps.

Source: Lin L., Vicente K.J., Doyle D.J.: Patient safety, potential adverse drug events, and medical device design: A human factors engineering approach. *J Biomed Inform* 34:274–284, Aug. 2001. Used with permission.

with the nurses and nursing students showed that an overwhelming majority (100% of nursing students and 90% of nurses) preferred the programming interface of the redesigned pump.

Collectively, the findings of this study show that measurable improvements in equipment safety and efficiency can be achieved by adopting a human factors approach to interface design. The study also illustrates a template for conducting comparative usability tests before purchasing equipment.

Code Cart Design

At St. Mark's Hospital in Salt Lake City, a committee overseeing problems associated with codes was contemplating solutions to the cluttered and disorganized medication drawers of crash carts that were hindering retrieval of drugs. The project was initiated when a nurse who had recently learned about usability testing at a conference made the suggestion to apply usability testing to help them develop a solution.

Analysis

The project began by identifying the users and their tasks. The users of crash cart medication drawers were identified as experienced progressive care unit nurses with advanced cardiac life support (ACLS) certification and ICU training. The task was identifying vials, ampoules, and pre-filled syringes and preparing intravenous (IV) drugs for rapid administration. Current use of the code cart drug drawers was determined by reviewing the hospital's most recent 100 codes. This helped to establish the most frequently used drugs which should be included in the drawer. The ACLS guidelines were also consulted to determine if there were any missing or extraneous drugs.

To determine the baseline with the existing drug drawer (Figure 2-7, below), nurses were timed as they retrieved medications out of the drawer in a simulated code. Observations of the nurses were made as they searched for medications. On average, the task of identifying and removing the correct drug took 3:07 (minutes: seconds), which demonstrated a dire need for improving the drawer design.

Design

Next, work began on a prototype of a redesigned drawer. The first prototype had a rectangular piece of neutral colored foam with spaces cut out to fit ampules and vials. Drugs were placed in alphabetical order (although this has been shown to be error prone because drug names are often similar to one another, leading to the look-alike, sound-alike problem).[35]

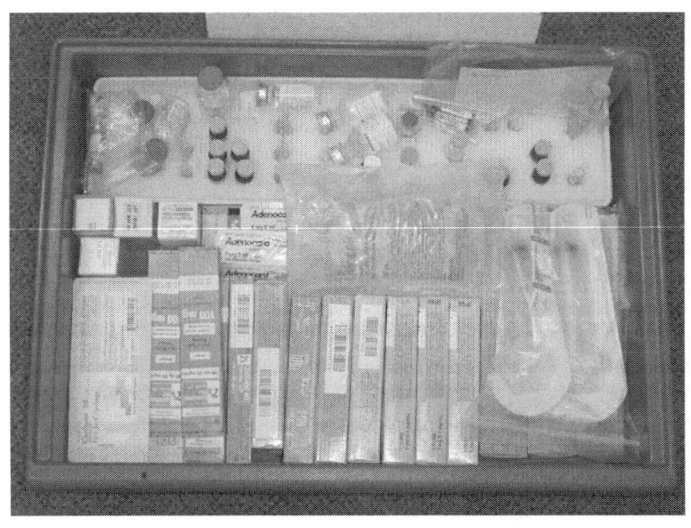

Figure 2-7. Existing Crash Cart Drawer

The existing crash cart is shown.

Source: McLaughlin R.C.: Redesigning the crash cart: Usability testing improves one facility's medication drawers. *Am J Nurs* 103:64A–64F, Apr. 2003. Used with permission.

CHAPTER 2
Methods and Tools

Testing

Usability tests were conducted with this prototype, and retrieval time was reduced to an average of 1:28. However, movement of the drawer caused shuffling of other medications, obscuring the vials. A second prototype was developed in which (1) a thicker foam block was used to prevent this shuffling, and (2) navy-colored foam was used to add contrast to aid vial recognition. Usability testing was then conducted, which yielded a further reduction in retrieval time. Ultimately, five prototypes were developed and tested, yielding an improved average retrieval time of 1:08. Each prototype tested different variations (labels on the foam block, different orientation of the labels, and so forth). The final test involved inserting a wrong medication in a labeled slot. The misplaced medication caused misidentification by one nurse who had read the label on the foam block instead of the vial. Other nurses took longer to retrieve medications from that prototype because they were now reading both the foam block label and the vial label.

Final Design

The final proposed design (Figure 2-8, below) included a foam platform that was raised to prevent shuffling within the drawer, a dark-colored background to facilitate recognition of the vials, and unlabeled slots for vials. The medications were all oriented so as to present the text on the labels horizontally (no longer requiring tilting of the head to read labels).

This example illustrates how usability testing and an iterative process helped to redesign crash carts. The result was measurable improvements in the time to retrieve drugs. If you are creating new solutions or improvements in your health

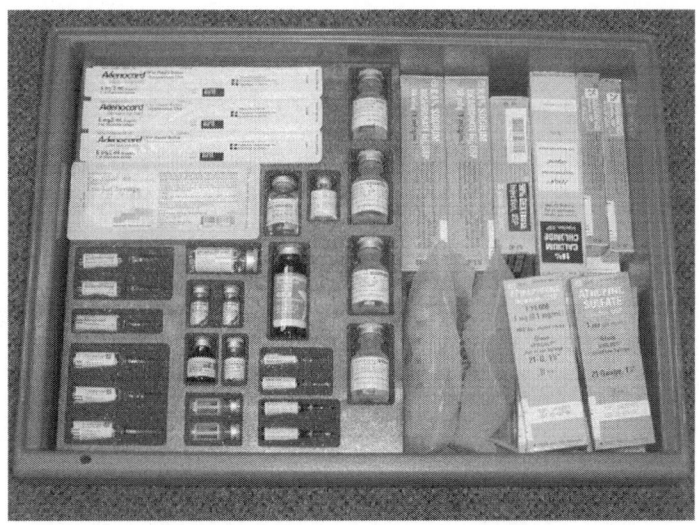

Figure 2-8. Final Redesign of the Crash Cart Drawer

The final redesign of the redesigned crash cart drawer is shown.

Source: McLaughlin R.C.: Redesigning the crash cart: Usability testing improves one facility's medication drawers. *Am J Nurs* 103:64A–64F, Apr. 2003. Used with permission.

care organization, this example illustrates how you can adopt an iterative process and usability testing to develop effective solutions.

Congestive Heart Failure (CHF) Order Sets
Multiple Redesign

In 2000, Advocate Christ Medical Center, a suburban tertiary care hospital in Oak Lawn, Illinois, sought to improve the care of patients with CHF.[36] Its cardiology division redesigned CHF order sets to increase their use (baseline was at 13%). The resulting standardized physician order sets—predetermined collections of orders which are departmentally sanctioned—were intended to promote efficiency and safety through compliance with clinical practice guidelines.

The order sets underwent another redesign in 2003, again primarily conducted by the cardiology division but this time with more physician feedback. To encourage change in physician behavior, the hospital management team employed quality improvement strategies such as offering in-service lectures by local and national experts on the management of CHF, issuing memos by the emergency department chair and the quality improvement chair, and posting signage and reminders to use the order sets. Yet these efforts failed: Order set use for eligible patients was at only 8%.

Recognizing that specific design elements of the order sets could contribute to an increase in compliance, the hospital decided in 2004 to use HFE to improve the order sets and embarked on a study to evaluate the impact of the human factors–based redesign on order set use and compliance with clinical practice guidelines.

The original CHF order set was not designed with usability in mind. It was unnecessarily complex (two pages long), provided multiple medication choices, and lacked organization. The new order set was more succinct and better organized and included narrative information to encourage use of clinical practice guidelines.

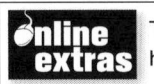 The order sets are provided online at http:/www.jcrinc.com/UHFE10/extras.

Testing

To evaluate usage, a descriptive retrospective medical record review of adult patients admitted from the emergency department with the primary diagnosis of CHF was conducted. Data were collected on acuity and clinical practice guideline parameters for 84 patients admitted before and 87 patients admitted after the introduction of the new CHF order set.

There was a significant increase in order set use by the first postintervention interval (POST). By the third POST, order set use reached 72%, compared to the baseline of 9%. Paper-based products such as order sets often do not come to mind when identifying safety improvement projects. Yet, as this example illustrates, HFE can be applied to the design of low-technology products such as paper order forms and can have a stronger influence on human behavior than simply disseminating the order sets and providing training and memos. The compliance with clinical practice guidelines and use of the order sets was improved through the use of HFE in the design.

CONCLUSION

In addition to a knowledge base about human characteristics and human performance, HFE brings tools and methods that can help health care organizations in their patient safety activities. This chapter introduced a small subset of those methods and tools. For health care organizations that want to learn more about or begin to implement some of these methods and tools, it is highly recommended that they refer to the case study examples in Chapters 5–10.

Also, the Appendix (pages 71–75) presents many references that cannot usually be found in one place.

References

1. Bias R.G., Mayhew D.J.: *Cost-Justifying Usability: An Update for the Internet Age,* 2nd ed. San Francisco: Morgan Kaufmann Publishers, 2005.
2. Martin J.L: Medical device development: The challenge for ergonomics. *Appl Ergon* 39:271–283, May 2008, Epub Dec. 3, 2007.
3. American National Standards Institute (ANSI)/Association for the Advancement of Medical Instrumentation (AAMI): *Human Factors Engineering: Design of Medical Devices.* (AAMI HE75:2009). Arlington, VA: AAMI, 2009.
4. Wiklund M.E., Wilcox S.B.: *Designing Usability into Medical Products.* Boca Raton, FL: CRC Press, 2004.
5. Miletello L.: A cognitive task analysis of NICU nurses' patient assessment skills. In *Proceedings of the 39th Annual Meeting of the Human Factors and Ergonomics Society.* San Diego: Human Factors and Ergonomics Society, 1995, pp. 733–737.
6. Shachak A., et al.: Primary care physicians' use of an electronic medical record system: a cognitive task analysis *J Gen Intern Med* 4:341–334 Mar. 2009.
7. Peyre S.E., et al.: Laparoscopic Nissen fundoplication assessment: Task analysis as a model for the development of a procedural checklist. *Surg Endosc* 26:1227–1232, Jun. 2009.
8. Vicente K.J.: *Cognitive Work Analysis: Toward Safe, Productive, and Healthy Computer-Based Work.* Mahwah, NJ: Erlbaum and Associates, 1999.
9. Sharp T.D., Helmicki A.J.: The application of the ecological interface design approach to neonatal intensive care medicine. In *Proceedings of the 42nd Annual Meeting of the Human Factors and Ergonomics Society.* San Diego: Human Factors and Ergonomics Society, 1998, pp. 350–354.
10. Hajdukiewicz J.R., et al.: Modeling a medical environment: An ontology for integrated medical informatics design. *Int J Med Inform* 62:79–99, Jun. 2001.
11. Nielsen J.: *Usability Engineering.* Boston: AP Professional, 1993.
12. Lin L., et al.: Applying human factors to the design of medical equipment: Patient-controlled analgesia. *J Clin Monit Comput* 14:253–263, May 1998.
13. Carvalho C.J., Borycki E.M., Kushniruk A.W.: Using heuristic evaluations to assess the safety of health information systems. *Stud Health Technol Inform* 143:297–301, 2009.
14. Joshi A., et al.: Usability of a patient education and motivation tool using heuristic evaluation. *J Med Internet Res* 11:e47, Nov. 2009.
15. Chiu C.C., et al.: Usability assessment of pacemaker programmers. *Pacing Clin Electrophysiol* 27:1388–1398, Oct. 2004.
16. Graham M.J., et al.: Heuristic evaluation of infusion pumps: Implications for patient safety in intensive care units. *Int J Med Inform* 73:771–779, Nov. 2004.
17. Tang Z., et al.: Applying heuristic evaluation to improve the usability of a telemedicine system. *Telemed J E Health* 12:24–34, Feb. 2006.
18. Gosbee J.W.: The discovery phase of medical device design: A blend of intuition, creativity, and science. *Medical Device and Diagnostic Industry* 11:79–82, Nov. 1997.
19. Beyer H., Holtzblatt K.: *Contextual Design: Defining Customer-Centered Systems.* San Diego: Academic Press, 1998.
20. Brown D.S.: The challenges of a user-based design in a medical equipment market. In Wixon D., Ramey J. (eds.): *Field Methods Casebook for Software Design.* New York City: John Wiley & Sons, 1996, pp. 157–176.
21. Coble J.M., et al.: Contextual inquiry: Discovering physicians' true needs. *Proc Annu Symp Comput Appl Med Care,* pp. 469–473, 1995.
22. Blechner M., et al.: Using contextual design to identify potential innovations for problem based learning. *AMIA Annu Symp Proc.* 2003. http://www.ncbi.nlm.nih.gov/pmc/articles/PMC1479946 (accessed May 18, 2010).
23. Rubin J.J., Chisnell D.: *Handbook of Usability Testing: How to Plan, Design, and Conduct Effective Tests,* 2nd ed. Indianapolis: Wiley, 2008.
24. Garmer K., Ylvén J., Karlsson I.C.M.: User participation in requirements elicitation comparing focus group interviews and usability tests for eliciting usability requirements for medical equipment: A case study. *Int J Ind Ergon* 33:85–98, Feb. 2004.
25. McLaughlin R.C.: Redesigning the crash cart: Usability testing improves one facility's medication drawers. *Am J Nurs* 103:64A–64F, Apr. 2003.
26. Lin L., Vicente K.J., Doyle D.J.: Patient safety, potential adverse drug events, and medical device design: A human factors engineering approach. *J Biomed Inform* 34:274–284, Aug. 2001.
27. Merry A.F., et al.: A simulation design for research evaluating safety innovations in anaesthesia. *Anaesthesia* 63:1349–1357, Dec. 2008.
28. Uzawa Y., Yamada Y., Suzukawa M.: Evaluation of the user interface simplicity in the modern generation of mechanical ventilators. *Respir Care* 53:329–337, Mar. 2008.
29. Vignaux L., Tassaux D., Jolliet P.: Evaluation of the user-friendliness of seven new generation intensive care ventilators. *Intensive Care Med* 35:1687–1691, Oct. 2009. Epub Jul. 29, 2009.
30. Diggory P., et al.: Comparison of elderly people's technique in using two dry powder inhalers to deliver zanamivir: Randomised controlled trial. *BMJ* 322(7286):577–579, Mar. 10, 2001.
31. Wolski C.A.: Engineering detectives: Using human factors engineering to evaluate medical equipment helps make devices safer and more effective. *24x7,* Sep. 2008. http://www.24x7mag.com/issues/articles/2008-09_02.asp (accessed Apr. 13, 2010).

32. Hamman W.R., et al.: Using in situ simulation to identify and resolve latent environmental threats to patient safety: Case study involving a labor and delivery ward. *J Patient Saf* 5:184–187, Sep. 2009.
33. Kantner L., Sova D.H., Rosenbaum S.: Alternative methods for field usability research. *Proceedings of the 21st Annual International Conference on Documentation*. New York City: Association for Computing Machinery pp. 68–72, 2003.
34. Gosbee L.L.: Making patients safer: The human factor. Grand Rounds Lecture. Sunnybrook and Women's Health Science Centre. Toronto, Sep. 30, 2004.
35. U.S. Pharmacopeia: Look-alike/sound-alike drug products affect cognition. *Patient Safety CAPSLink*™, May 2004. http://www.usp.org/pdf/EN/patientSafety/capsLink2004-05-01.pdf (accessed Apr. 11, 2010).
36. Reingold S., Kulstad E.: Impact of human factor design on the use of order sets in the treatment of congestive heart failure. *Acad Emerg Med* 14:1097–1105, Nov. 2007.

CHAPTER 3

Lessons Learned in Teaching Human Factors Engineering

John W. Gosbee, M.D., M.S.; Laura Lin Gosbee, M.A.Sc.

Early in my career as an human factors engineering (HFE) consultant [J.W.G.], I was hired to do an HFE analysis of intravenous (IV) fluid and medication mixing in a hospital's pharmacy. The analysis included many hours of observation and contextual inquiry (Chapter 2). The overall goal was to look at the design of the mixing systems to identify areas with HFE flaws. During one observation, I was watching pharmacists and pharmacy technicians as they moved around the area of the main hospital pharmacy in conducting the tasks involved in the preparation of IV fluids and medications. Earlier that day, the pharmacy manager had given me a lengthy tour as he showed me the steps that represented the "day in the life" of IV medications—from the loading dock to disposal. He strongly suggested that I spend my time near the IV fluid mixing counter (that is, the hood), where I was most likely to encounter HFE problems.

I watched a pharmacist frantically type information into a desktop computer for 20 minutes and then, suddenly picking up a paper form, roll her stool over to a laptop computer. This laptop computer was in a fixed location and was attached to an IV fluid mixing device. The laptop was used only to run the mixing device. After typing for a minute or two, the pharmacist stopped, cursed, and hit the countertop with her hand. After staring at the computer screen for a minute, she again looked at the paper form on the counter and began slowly typing. Soon, when she seemed to have finished, she rolled the stool back to the desktop computer to resume her frantically paced typing. After 10 minutes, she took another paper form and rolled over to the laptop, hit a few buttons, yelled, and started swearing again.

After she calmed down, I walked over to ask her what was it about the laptop computer that was causing her such frustration. She muttered something about its role in calculating amounts of various stock fluids needed for total parenteral nutrition orders, exclaiming, "I must be the stupidest person to keep typing the wrong key and then having to reenter all the numbers on this screen." It was then that I remarked on the label affixed to the top of the laptop screen, which stated, "Do not hit the 'Enter' key to enter data, use the space bar." "Yes," she continued, "this reminder sign is supposed to keep me from using this laptop program like my desktop computer programs, where I use the 'Enter' key." As the conversation continued, I was to find out that the customized system on the laptop computer was programmed using a database with the now odd convention of using spacebar to enter data—and that using the "Enter" key instead wiped out all the data. Apparently, there was no way for either the hospital or vendor to reprogram the computer without redoing the system entirely. We agreed that it was fortunate that hitting the more logical "Enter" key did not cause a worse malfunction.

This interaction taught me several things—"nuggets"—about the practice of HFE in real-life settings. First, well-meaning clinical experts may not have complete insight into the where and how certain HFE issues may be found. Second, an HFE professional could use swearing and fist-pounding as signs of HFE issues to look deeper into. Third, interviews or questionnaires will miss many HFE issues when the people involved blame themselves.

In our combined 28 years of doing HFE analysis in home care, ambulatory care, and hospital settings, we have gathered practical nuggets like the ones that arose from the hospital pharmacy project. We have found that these practical tips are necessary, even for HFE professionals, because design hazards cannot easily be seen otherwise. Another finding is that many people who toil with poorly designed work places or tools are *excited* to learn about and employ HFE. Sidebar 3-1 (below) describes the "top 10" pearls that we have found useful for doing the "practice" of HFE. To use a medical analogy, they are like "clinical pearls." Most of these pearls include a strong element of teaching and persuading. Pearl 10 provides insight into one method that is useful to change a clinician's or manager's mind-set.

Sidebar 3-1. Top 10 Pearls of Conducting a Human Factors Engineering (HFE) Practice in Health Care

1. Draw on patients' experiences and comments to identify HFE issues, such as those related to medical devices, medication labeling and delivery systems, and information systems (that interact directly with them).[1]

2. To identify device-related HFE issues, ask biomedical or clinical engineers which devices do nurses and physicians label as "broken" even if "nothing" can be found wrong with them.[2]

3. Ask nurse and clinical educators which devices generate confusion in in-service training sessions—where the training does not seem to "stick." (The educators may find themselves saying, "Why doesn't this training help?" or "Why are our technicians and doctors so stupid?")

4. While in a hospital, a clinic, or any other setting, keep your ears tuned for people swearing when using devices or software or for phrases such as, "What is it doing?" or "Why is it doing that?"

5. Try to always use a heuristic evaluation (as described in Chapter 2) checklist when reviewing work areas, tools, and software. This cognitive aid decreases the chance of missing HFE issues. An example of a heuristic evaluation tool is provided in Sidebar 3-2 (page 58). Heuristic evaluation questions can also be

(continued)

Sidebar 3-1. Top 10 Pearls of Conducting a Human Factors Engineering (HFE) Practice in Health Care (continued)

adapted for specific types of devices by searching the HFE literature in a specific area, such as IV pumps.[3]

6. To identify HFE issues with devices and software in home care or care of patients with chronic conditions, ask patient educators—for example, diabetes nurses are likely to be familiar with patients' experiences with glucometers,[4] or nurses who work with patients with allergies would know about HFE issues related to epinephrine auto-injectors.

7. *Always* visit and observe for yourself; never assume anything regarding the nature and depth of HFE issues, no matter how much you think you know about a setting, device, or process. Missing an HFE "diagnosis" by not observing is just as likely as missing a clinical diagnosis by not doing a history and physical examination.

8. Keep a sharp eye for sticky notes, after-market signs and labels, or other telltale HFE clues when you visit and observe a clinical work area. If someone has paid, for example, for a professional-looking engraved plastic sign to be permanently affixed to a device or computer monitor, you have to assume a catastrophic HFE design issue until proved otherwise.

9. Provide workshops and on-the-job training during projects for clinicians and frontline managers to learn how HFE knowledge and skills can help them protect patients and be better physicians, nurses, pharmacists, and so on.

10. Use hands-on demonstrations to prompt clinicians and other health care personnel to "bend" their thinking toward HFE.[5] This is useful, for example, when "warming up" a root cause analysis team or for more in-depth workshops (as mentioned in Pearl 9).

References
1. Gosbee L.L.: Nuts! I can't figure out how to use my life-saving epinephrine auto-injector! *Jt Comm J Qual Saf* 30:220–223, Apr. 2004.
2. Draper S., Nielsen G.A., Noland M.: Using "no problem found" in infusion pump programming as a springboard for learning about human factors engineering. *Jt Comm J Qual Saf* 30:515–520, Sep. 2004.
3. Graham M.J., et al.: Heuristic evaluation of infusion pumps: Implications for patient safety in intensive care units. *Int J Med Inform* 73:771–779, Nov. 2004.
4. Rogers W.A., et al.: Analysis of a "simple" medical device. *Ergonomics in Design* 9:9, Winter 2001. http://www.hfes.org/web/Newsroom/Winter01EIDarticle1.pdf (accessed Mar. 26, 2010).
5. Gosbee J., Anderson T.: Human factors engineering design demonstrations can enlighten your RCA team. *Qual Saf Health Care* 12:119–121, Apr. 2003.

Source: Adapted from Gosbee J.W., Gosbee L.L.: *Pearls of HFE Practice in Healthcare*. Ann Arbor, MI: Red Forest Consulting, 2009. ©2009 Red Forest Consulting.

Sidebar 3-2. Heuristic Evaluation Tool: Getting Started

Product Metaphor
- Is it obvious what the device is at a glance?
- Is it obvious how to use it at a glance?
- Does the device work the same way as previous models or similar brands? Does this help or hinder the user?
- Does the device look like another device? Is that helpful in telling the user how to use it?
- Is the name of the device helpful in telling the user what it is, or how it's used?

Feedback and Displayed Messages
- Is it easy to tell what the device is doing at any given moment?
- When completing a task, is it obvious when you are successful vs. unsuccessful?
- At any given point in operating the device, can you tell exactly what you need to do next?
- If you hand the device to someone, can they figure where you've left off and what they need to do next?
- Can you understand the meaning of messages, symbols, sounds, or lights that are displayed?

Functionality of Controls
- Is it obvious what each button, dial, or switch will do?
- Are the controls grouped in a logical and helpful manner?
- Are the primary controls located in a way that makes them easy to access and operate?
- Do buttons look like buttons?
- Do any nonfunctional features of the device look like buttons or controls?
- Are critical controls differentiated from other controls?
- Does the size or shape of the buttons, dials, or switches make them difficult to use?

Labels and Warnings
- Can you easily see all the important labels and warnings?
- Are they located in an appropriate and relevant spot?
- Are the warning labels legible?
- Is the language understandable? Symbols meaningful? Or is special knowledge needed to interpret it?
- Do any labels obscure critical controls, lights, or parts of the device?
- Do any labels create visual clutter that might cause confusion?

Source: Red Forest Consulting. Used with permission.

The remainder of this chapter further addresses the preparation and delivery of HFE teaching in health care.

TEACHING HFE MIND-SET AND PRACTICE

HFE workshops are one of the most requested activities when doing HFE consulting for health care organizations and academia. The reason why is that they represent a familiar activity to help introduce participants to a new mind-set and practice. The learning objectives for various groups will differ, as follows:
- Medical students are trying to integrate HFE with clinical content, such as anatomy and emergency care of patients with acute abdominal pain.
- Patient safety specialists are seeking a complementary role for HFE, along with their quality improvement tools and event-investigation activities, such as root cause analysis (RCA).
- Managers and supervisors want to know how HFE can help them promote the "safety culture," and, hopefully, help the organization identify lasting remedies that go beyond more training and new policies.

Teaching HFE to Trainees

Teaching HFE to medical students and residents has been a career-long quest for us.[1,2] In my [J.W.G.] work at University of Michigan Medical School and other medical schools, I have created HFE learning objectives for trainees, who have ranged from first-year medical students to full professors. The common goals have been to create practitioners who would be more *valuable* and active *partners* in redesigning devices, workspaces, and software to reduce the risk of patient harm.

In teaching trainees systems thinking, which forms the basis for HFE mind-set and tools, I encourage trainees to also use it in diagnosis and treatment aspects of patient-centered care. For example, when the fourth-year medical student is applying HFE in redesigning a form to guide the patient's preparation for colonoscopy, he is also learning to anticipate the information needs, beliefs, and common misunderstandings of the thousands of patients he will eventually see in his or her future gastrointestinal practice.

Medical schools, teaching hospitals, and other organizations are increasingly addressing patient safety, including implicit or explicit HFE objectives and content, in their curricula. The effort to develop patient safety curricula has been given a recent boost by the Lucian Leape Institute report *Unmet Needs: Teaching Physicians to Provide Safe Patient Care,* which indicates to "practice safely, and to improve care, students need to learn safety science, human factors engineering concepts, systems thinking, and the science of improvement."[3] For example, the World Health Organization's (WHO) *Patient Safety Curriculum Guide for Medical Schools* lists the following HFE objectives[4]:
- Explain the meaning of the term *human factors.*
- Explain the relationship between human factors and patient safety.
- Apply human factors thinking to their work environment.

Sidebar 3-3 (page 60) provides an outline of a faculty-development workshop that I provided for a large academic medical center, which wanted to address physician teachers' and senior residents' interest in patient safety. The rationale was that the workshop would inform not only the attendees' daily clinical practice but also their supervision of medical students and residents. Many sessions in the workshop were not primarily focused on HFE, but all the sessions were organized to deliver the message that redesign is needed to give clinicians the best possible chance of success.

Sidebar 3-3. Learning Objectives and Agenda for a Three-Day Patient Safety and HFE Workshop

Objectives
1. Know the theoretical & practical reasons why "blame and train" approaches fail.
2. Become familiar with the basics of safety and human factors engineering.
3. Understand importance of discovering root causes toward developing proper interventions.
4. Become familiar with human factors engineering techniques that determine root causes and how this is crucial to the design of effective interventions.

Agenda (Three separate four-hour sessions)
DAY 1
Patient safety "diagnosis"
- Tips and tools to instill systems thinking—away from typical blame and shame
- Exercises to show that "violation" of policy is a symptom—not a diagnosis
- Role of these tools within morbidity and mortality conferences (M&Ms) and root cause analyses (RCAs)

Human factors engineering ("diagnosis" and "treatment")
- "Basic science" underlying patient safety concepts
- Practical tools to understand broken systems

DAY 2
Safety analysis tools that are usable and useful
- Cause-and-effect diagramming and Five Principles of Causation
- Using the tools during case conferences and M&Ms

Evidence-based patient safety ("treatment")
- Concepts and evidence behind stronger and weaker interventions
- Exercises to teach the concepts and tools
- Effectiveness of these concepts for guiding resident's safety projects

DAY 3
Successful formats for teaching patient safety (tools and tips), with in-depth focus on the following:
- Patient safety case conference (e.g., M&M)
- Class demonstrations and role play
- Patient safety on working rounds
- Patient safety projects (creating learning and lasting impact)

Curriculum program development
- Starting and sustaining your efforts
- Assessment tools to track resident's progress and your program's

Source: Red Forest Consulting. Used with permission.

CHAPTER 3
Lessons Learned in Teaching Human Factors Engineering

Teaching HFE to Clinicians

Teaching HFE to practicing nurses, physicians, and other clinicians can support larger HFE redesign efforts under way and increase reporting of HFE–related issues. HFE "spinoffs" of ongoing assessment and improvement activities, such as RCAs, can also be conducted. For example, an RCA team at an academic medical center was investigating an event of a retained sponge following a surgical procedure. Early on, the team focused on the specific failings of the surgical nurse and on outdated policies. The patient safety manager provided hands-on HFE design demonstrations to redirect the RCA team's focus from training or policies to design-related issues that contributed to the event. The RCA team was then able to see design problems in the operating room and radiology information systems that heavily contributed to the sponge being missed.[5]

At the request of a large hospital system, which was undertaking a systemwide HFE project, I conducted a workshop and two teleconferences to establish and help the hospital system sustain an HFE analysis effort in the perioperative setting. The two four-hour workshop sessions were separated by a few weeks to provide an opportunity for the 40 participants to do their HFE homework and conduct an HFE "mini-project." The participants included physicians, nurses, and technicians from perioperative and intraoperative settings, as well as education and safety managers and leaders who wanted to apply HFE knowledge and skills to future projects. The workshop objectives and agenda are shown in Sidebar 3-4 (page 62). The teleconferences provided support for attendees in completing their homework and beginning their projects. In these teleconferences, I provided any midcourse correction for the projects, such as remembering to look up and apply pertinent human factors standards and to focus more on physical redesign and less on adding warning labels. I also sought feedback on how I should focus the curriculum for the second workshop session.

Teaching HFE to Leadership

A large university hospital requested an HFE workshop for hundreds of managers and supervisors from all over their integrated health system. The goal of the workshop was to balance the content of previous patient safety workshops on patient safety culture, team training, and other people-level fixes with a focus on redesign of devices, workspaces, and software. The objectives and agenda were similar to those of the workshop for frontline clinicians and safety managers and leaders, as described in the previous section. However, we also included (1) demonstrations and small-group exercises that provided more linkages to the types of undetected safety problems that these leaders might encounter and (2) activities, such as redesign of devices and workspaces, to highlight the value of HFE.

The exercises enabled the attendees to practice detecting design issues with everyday items, such as a stove-top layout (Figure 3-1, page 63). In this exercise, most attendees can humorously recall turning on the wrong burner due to this design flaw, even on a stove they have used for years. In the moment of this chagrin, the attendees are then asked to think about medical device or health care software examples of this kind of control-display confusion.

In the workshop, group redesign practice continues with medical devices whose clinical use is easily understood by nonexpert users. Using these type of examples is key because many managers or leaders may not be clinicians or may have not done clinical work for a while. One example is the confusing display of an insulin-injection pen, whose display can be read upside down (Figure 3-2, page 64). The audi-

Sidebar 3-4. Learning Objectives and Agenda for a Two-Day (with Interim Period) Human Factors Engineering (HFE) Workshop

Objectives
1. Gain an understanding of HFE as applied to health care and patient safety.
2. Attain skills in HFE analysis and practice applying to redesign of forms, devices, and work areas—with focus on perioperative and intraoperative systems.
3. Attain skills in the HFE method of usability testing and fitting it into proactive risk assessment of correct-site surgery.

Agendas
DAY ONE
- HFE overview and demonstrations of key concepts
- Usability testing group demonstrations
- Usability testing small-group exercise with medical device(s)
- Redesign with devices (e.g., AED)
- Redesign practice continues as applied to work area (pediatric hospital room)
- Mentored small groups develop test plan for assigned project

INTERIM
- Apply heuristic evaluation and then redesign oxygen cylinder regulator to decrease confusion about full versus empty
- Observe and do heuristic evaluation on a device, software screen, or work area in surgery-related settings

DAY TWO
- Usability testing of an actual device
- Applying HFE to processes and policies (designing to improve patient safety practices)
- Inventive problem solving using TRIZ*
- Lessons from homework and projects
- Learning how to apply HFE to your "next" safety issue (small group)
- Learning where to find "hidden" HFE information, publications, and other useful resources

AED, automated external defibrillator. *TRIZ, Teoriya Resheniya Izobretatelskikh Zadatch* (Russian acronym for "The Theory of Inventive Problem Solving," developed by Genrikh Altshuller and colleagues, beginning in 1946).

* Gosbee J.W.: Use of problem-solving tools of TRIZ to address equipment design for home care. In Winters J.M., Story M.F. (eds.): *Accessibility and Usability Considerations for Medical Instrumentation.* New York City: CRC Press, 2006, pp. 271–282.

Source: Red Forest Consulting. Used with permission.

CHAPTER 3
Lessons Learned in Teaching Human Factors Engineering

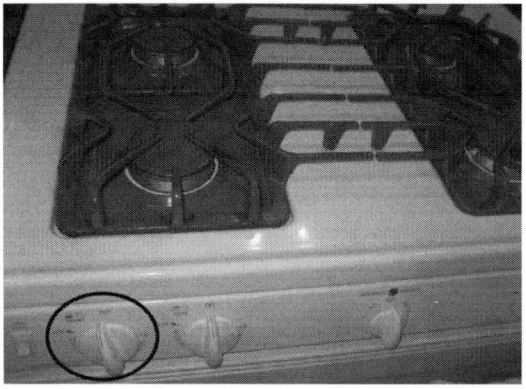

Figure 3-1. Stove-Top Burner Picture for Group Exercise

In the stove-top burner exercise, the task is to identify which burner is controlled by the knob on the left (circled)—the answer is the back burner.

Source: Red Forest Consulting. Used with permission.

ence is asked to think about what each display is indicating, and a surprising number have to be told, and are shocked to find, that the insulin-containing pen is so easy to misread.

Then the audience is asked to think about the design reasons for confusion and how to redesign a pen with more "up-ness" and "down-ness." Some of the attendees will simply say that patients need to be trained or be warned about this possible misstep Many others will offer stronger solutions, such as using higher-resolution displays, underlining the numbers, or widening the display and putting the label "Units" after the numbers (Figure 3-3, page 65). A few will suggest more invasive redesign, such as flattening one side of the pen to make it feel more like the bottom or turning the display by 90 degrees. If the display is turned, the user is more likely to hold the nondisplay part of the pen in the correct orientation. The kind of lively discussion that ensues helps the attendees recognize the commonality of such design-induced confusion.

We explicitly address the fact that most of the managers and leaders will not have the ability to change the design of devices or other medical hardware. However, we emphasize that they can use their knowledge of HFE flaws in purchasing the next version of a device, customizing training, and designing cognitive aids such as mini–user guides. Yet we do include redesign exercises for situations in which they might have more control, such as reorganizing furniture and permanent storage (for example, cabinets) and work surfaces (countertops) in a hospital room to reduce any inadvertent contamination between dirty and clean items.

In addition to the more applicable exercises, we provide examples in which researchers have simply redesigned paper and computer forms to improve usage and safety—such as the HFE redesign of a congestive heart failure standard

Figure 3-2. Insulin Pens

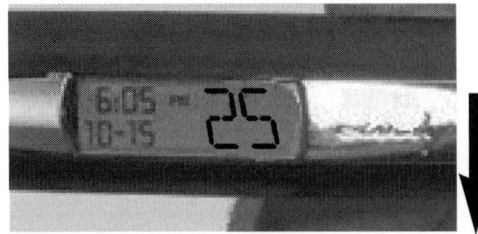 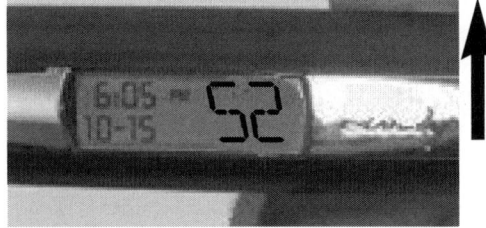

The displays on two insulin pens are shown; the pen on the left is upside down.

order form, which increased physician usage from 9% to 72%,[6] as mentioned in Chapter 2. In a recent study, researchers found that by redesigning the seemingly innocuous boldfaced "epinephrine" in a bradycardia algorithm on an emergency reminder card by removing the boldfacing, the number of code teams that incorrectly chose epinephrine as the first-line medication in simulated emergency scenarios decreased from 12.2% to 2.4%.[7]

TOP FIVE PEARLS OF TEACHING HFE

We now provide our "top five" pearls of teaching HFE to health care audiences.

1. HFE is a "high-contact sport." The first goal is to "flip people's brains around 180 degrees," whether the trainees are, as we stated earlier, first-year medical students or full professors.

2. Become interactive or die! Adult learning theory is many decades old, and even most continuing medical education departments know that podium-bound teachers' lecturing is often not the most effective form of instruction. In a four-hour workshop, we include at least two hours of hands-on, small-group work—and approximately five hours in a full-day workshop.

3. If hands-on, small-group exercises are useful, allowing groups to innovate and redesign is even better. For example, in providing device and architecture-type HFE exercises, we have found that workshop attendees have often refused to stop working and take their break.[8]

4. Be able to "scale down." Have some interactive "demos" that fit in your pocket and take seconds to do with a few people—such as an insulin pen (trainer) that is harder to use and an insulin pen that is easier to use. The best HFE examples are ones that you found in your organization and addressed. These HFE demos are useful in selling the idea of HFE's uniqueness to a wide range of audiences—from a small group struggling to innovate on stubborn patient safety problems such as nonlabeled specimens to a vice president of patient safety with the budget authority to start a half-million dollar project.

5. It is better to start with and emphasize more complex examples, such as those that are based on "holistic" HFE research rather than, say, medical device–related issues. For example, we recently found that even in an introductory workshop, most of the attendees (clinicians) found that HFE analysis of a complicated system behind thoracostomy[9] was more instructive than that of an insulin pen. Clinicians do not usually view the familiar procedure of thoracos-

CHAPTER 3
Lessons Learned in Teaching Human Factors Engineering

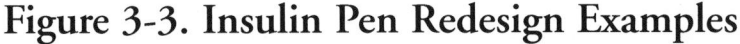

Figure 3-3. Insulin Pen Redesign Examples

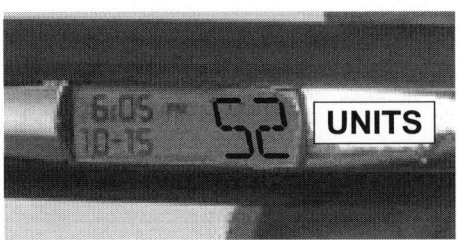
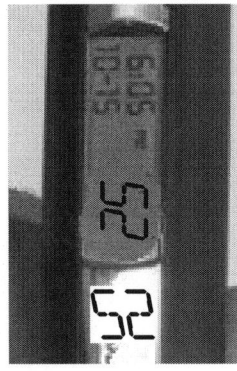

Redesign examples include widening the display and putting the label "Units" after the numbers (left) or turning the display by 90 degrees (right).

tomy to be complex, whereas HFE professionals are likely to see it as massively complex.

SUMMARY

Learning about HFE concepts and methods is not sufficient to qualify someone to practice HFE in a health care setting. The top 10 pearls in Table 3-1 reveal many of the less obvious ways we have learned to find and help solve HFE problems in our complex health care settings. Because teaching and persuading decision makers and allied clinicians is a big part of HFE "practice," we have provided sample agendas, exercises, and ways to make HFE professionals' teaching and efforts at persuasion more effective.

References

1. Stahlhut R.W., Gosbee J.W.: A human-centered approach to medical informatics for medical students, residents, and practicing clinicians. *Acad Med* 72:881–887, Oct. 1997
2. Gosbee J.W.: Use of problem-solving tools of TRIZ to address equipment design for home care. In Winters J.M., Story M.F. (eds.): *Accessibility and Usability Considerations for Medical Instrumentation.* New York City: CRC Press, 2006, pp. 271–282.
3. National Patient Safety Foundation: "New Lucian Leape Institute Report Finds That U.S. Medical Schools Are Falling Short in Teaching Physicians about how to Provide Safe Patient Care" (news release). http://www.npsf.org/pr/pressrel/2010-03-10.php (accessed Mar. 2010).
4. World Health Organization (WHO): *WHO Patient Safety Curriculum Guide: WHO Patient Safety Curriculum Guide for Medical Schools.* Geneva, Switzerland, 2008. http://www.who.int/patientsafety/education/curriculum/en/index.html (accessed Mar. 26, 2010).
5. Gosbee J., Anderson T.: Human factors engineering design demonstrations can enlighten your RCA team. *Qual Saf Health Care* 12:119–121, Apr. 2003.
6. Reingold S., Kulstad E.: Impact of human factor design on the use of order sets in the treatment of congestive heart failure. *Acad Emerg Med* 14:1097–1105, Nov. 2007.
7. Cash P., Bunegin L., Sperduti A.: Does the AHA Bradycardia Algorithm encourage inadvertent administration of epinephrine during treatment of symptomatic bradycardia [abstract]. *Simulation in Healthcare* 4(4):307, 2009.
8. Gosbee L.L., Gosbee J.W: B*aby Jaws of Life: A Human Factors Engineering Workbook.* Ann Arbor, MI: Red Forest Consulting, 2007.
9. Seagull F.J., et al.: Video-based ergonomic analysis to evaluate thoracostomy tube placement techniques. *J Trauma* 60:227–232, Jan. 2006.

CHAPTER 4

Finding and Using Human Factors Engineering Expertise

Laura Lin Gosbee, M.A.Sc.; John W. Gosbee, M.D., M.S.

In this chapter, we talk about what a health care organization can look for when hiring a human factors engineering (HFE) professional.

FINDING THE HFE PROFESSIONAL "RIGHT" FOR THE ORGANIZATION

If HFE is new to your vocabulary and you have never worked with an HFE professional, you may be wondering, "What do I need to know to get on the pathway toward working with one?" Even more elementarily, how does a person become an HFE professional? Should he or she have a special degree or specialized training? How do I know what qualifications and skills to look for? Finally, you are probably asking a question that never shows up in print in any job search, "What should we avoid?"

How Does a Person Become an HFE Professional?

To become an HFE professional, the typical course of study is a human factors degree from a university offering such a program.* Many HFE professionals have a graduate degree, which will likely be in engineering or psychology—but their field of study is HFE, and their program will consist of human factors course work along with, typically, a thesis or research project. Persons who study engineering before entering a graduate HFE program (for example, industrial or systems engineering) often learn about the broader industrial engineering discipline that gave rise to not only human factors but the fields of quality and safety engineering, process improvement (for example, Lean and Six Sigma), and operations research (for example, logistics and scheduling). In addition to engineering, you may also find HFE professionals with an undergraduate degree in education, computer science, and, occasionally, anthropology, who have gone on to pursue a graduate degree in HFE.

Human factors programs may vary quite significantly from one another in terms of their course offerings. Therefore, students wishing to study human factors may select a program on the basis of their interest in a particular subspecialty or area of human factors (for instance, information processing and decision making in air traffic control). Sidebar 4-1 (page 69) lists the required and elective courses for graduate

---

* For a listing of graduate-level HFE programs, see Human Factors and Ergonomics Society: *Directory of Human Factors/Ergonomics Graduate Programs in the United States and Canada.* http://www.hfes.org/Web/Students/grad_programs.html (accessed Apr. 14, 2010). Similar information about programs in other countries is currently being assembled by the International Ergonomics Association: *Professional Standards and Education Committee.* http://www.iea.cc/browse.php?contID=professional_standards_education_committee_2 (accessed May 11, 2010)

programs in the United States and Canada. The Human Factors and Ergonomics Society provides information on the courses offered at the undergraduate and at each of the HFE graduate-level programs.[1,2]

Some master's degree programs involve only course work, while others may require extensive research projects or a thesis. The projects or thesis may focus on theoretical aspects of human factors, or it could be more applied in nature, depending on the interest of the student. Doctoral degree programs in HFE all require a thesis project or dissertation on an applied research topic.

There are also a limited number of human factors programs at the undergraduate level. One can find undergraduate degree programs focused on human factors[1] or industrial engineering programs with extensive HFE course offerings and practical projects.

Nine Tips on Hiring an HFE Professional

We have compiled a list of nine hiring tips to answer the final two questions, "How do I know what qualifications and skills to look for?" and "What should we avoid"? This list reflects (1) our direct experience in hiring such people for a university hospital and a patient safety organization, and (2) our indirect experience in helping hospitals, government agencies, and industry develop HFE programs (for example, job descriptions) and enact recruitment.

1. Consult with an HFE professional. If you do not have someone in your organization knowledgeable about HFE and its typical course of training, you may wish to consult with an HFE professional to help you narrow down the kinds of background and skill set that are desirable for your organization.

2. Learn about HFE specializations. Ask candidates to identify the specific areas in HFE in which they have been trained or schooled. You will want to see if their interests, training, and/or experience are in the same area(s) that you envision for HFE work in your organization. For example, if you envision them working with you to evaluate electronic devices and software systems, do they have course work/experience related to human-computer interaction, cognitive psychology, and/or human factors methods for evaluating usability? If you are more interested in preventing workplace injuries, do they have a background that includes occupational medicine?

3. Learn about their program. You can learn more about a candidate's HFE focus even before the interview by looking up the program(s) and school(s) he or she attended. Sometimes, you can look up the required course work in the program or identify the research interests of the faculty to see what area(s) of HFE is strongly supported in that program.

4. Seek candidates from programs with cross-trained teachers and interprofessional courses. Although only a few such programs exist, those that have faculty who are trained across disciplines or that offer interprofessional courses to allow students to *become* cross-trained (for example, an HFE program might include coursework in physiology or biomedical instrumentation) enable students to learn how to apply HFE principles and methods in the health care domain. Students who wish to pursue HFE but who are in programs without cross-trained faculty may wish to choose mentors or advisors from both the HFE department and a health care–related department or school (such as medical, nursing, biomedical engineering, or pharmacy). Medical professionals who go on to become HFE professionals (for example, the paramedic, nurse, physician, pharma-

> ## Sidebar 4-1. List of Required and Elective Courses for Graduate Programs in Human Factors (HF) and Ergonomics
>
> - Experimental Research Methods or Methods in HF
> - Statistics/Quantitative Methods/Design/Measurements
> - Foundations of HF/Applied Experimental/Applied Cognitive/Cognitive Engineering/Engineering Psychology
> - Sensation & Perception or Perception
> - Visual Science
> - Physiology/Biopsychology
> - Cognitive/Information Processing/Decision Making
> - Learning
> - Psychomotor Skills Learning/Skilled Performance
> - Ergonomics/Biomechanics
> - Social/Personality/Organizational/Individual Differences/Personnel Psychology
> - Developmental/Aging
> - History & Systems
> - Human-Technology Interaction/Systems
> - Environmental
> - Human Performance/Abilities
> - Aerospace
> - Software
> - Controls/Displays/Workplace Layout
> - Professional Issues/Problems
> - Teaching Practicum/Teaching
> - Behavioral Neuroscience
> - Research/Directed Independent Study
> - Thesis/Doctoral Dissertation
> - Conference & Workshop
> - Graduate Seminar
> - Training
> - Manufacturing
> - Simulations
> - Topics in HF
> - Industrial Engineering
> - Epidemiology
> - Usability
> - Internship
> - Safety/Safety Engineering
> - Physical Agents
> - Industrial Engineering Methods
> - Injury Prevention/Injuries
> - Health/Stress Issues
> - Occupational Medicine
> - Reliability
> - Carpal Tunnel Syndrome
> - Work Environment/Management
>
> **Source:** Human Factors and Ergonomics Society: *Human Factors/Ergonomics Courses Offered Across Programs.* http://www.hfes.org/Web/EducationalResources/coursesmain.html (accessed Apr. 14, 2010). Used with permission.

cist, or biomedical engineer who then earns an HFE degree)—or vice versa—are likely to be particularly promising (if rare) candidates. Such cross-training allows the HFE professional to have insight into the broad and varied nature of HFE applications in health care.

5. Find out about their projects. Ask candidates about the kind of HFE projects that they have led or have participated in as part of their current or previous positions or course work. Look for experience in working on the kinds of projects that you would envision them working on at your own organization—consider not just the topic area but their ability to participate in a multidisciplinary team, teach or give presentations (communication skills), write reports or grant applications, and manage their time with multiple projects. They should also have some level of ability to grasp technical aspects of the systems and technology used in health care.

6. Determine if they can tolerate a clinical setting. You are going to ask candidates to spend much of their time in a high-stress environment that may well entail the sight of blood and the smell of emesis. It would be ideal to find a candidate who has volunteered in a health care setting or has other similar frontline experience. In addition to tolerating the clinical work environment, the candidates would need to understand or be able to quickly learn the language, technology, science and other work-context characteristics of the clinical setting.

7. Consider their understanding of research methodology. Depending on their program of study, HFE candidates may or may not have had training in research methodology. Such training would enable them to understand study design and understand how to determine cause-and-effect relationships. This is an important factor if the HFE candidate is to be involved in patient safety research or is to conduct human factors testing or usability testing.

8. Passion beats credentials. Look for a candidate who has a passion for working in the health care domain. Has someone the candidate knew suffered an HFE–related adverse event? Did he or she forge a pathway into the health care domain at a time when few HFE practitioners were doing so? Affirmative responses to either of these questions likely means that such a candidate has a strong personal desire to work in the field and that he or she will likely make a better candidate than a less passionate one from a top-10 program. Because a good part of his or her job may deal with the sad and tragic consequences of adverse medical incidents, a candidate with this passion may be better prepared to overcome such stress.

9. Systems thinking and knowledge about the design process are essential. As with any scientific field, it is essential for an HFE professional to have the necessary theoretical knowledge. However, when it comes to developing long-lasting solutions to HFE problems in your health care organization, you need an HFE professional who can not only diagnose the problems using knowledge of HFE science but who can also apply systems thinking to develop a solution. In other words, you do *not* want an HFE candidate who responds to HFE–related problems with only training interventions, when most systems issues can and should be mitigated through design or redesign (fit the task/tool to the human, not the other way around)—Chapter 2 discusses the role of HFE methods in the design process.

In Chapters 5–10, authors from six different health care organizations recount how their organizations came to seek HFE expertise. These accounts, which are described from the perspective of the health care organization (Chapters 5 and 10) and the HFE professional (Chapters 6–9), illustrate the range of HFE issues being tackled and the varied roles that HFE professionals take on in these organizations. The case studies on HFE projects featured in the chapters address a broad range of topics, showcasing applications of HFE to improve safety and efficiency in health care.

References

1. Human Factors and Ergonomics Society: *Human Factors/Ergonomics Undergraduate Programs.* http://www.hfes.org/Web/Students/undergradprograms.html (accessed Apr. 14, 2010).
2. Human Factors and Ergonomics Society: *Human Factors/Ergonomics Courses Offered Across Programs.* http://www.hfes.org/Web/EducationalResources/coursesmain.html (accessed Apr. 14, 2010).

APPENDIX

Human Factors Engineering Resources

This Appendix lists a variety of human factors engineering (HFE) resources. The references are organized on the basis of different needs because books, articles, reports, and other resources on HFE vary widely in focus and depth. For example, if you are interested in justifying the creation of a usability laboratory at your health care organization, you may be interested in the sections "If you want to educate leadership about HFE in your health care organization" to help you build a business case and "If you want to get deeper" to gain an understanding of how to conduct usability tests. There are also references to guidance documents for the reader who is involved in a development project ("If you want guidance for a design project"). You will also find many more resources in other categories to help you get started on your road to learning more about HFE. (Note: All URLs are current as of publication date.)

If you have just begun to learn about HFE

Casey S.: *Set Phasers on Stun: And Other True Tales of Design, Technology, and Human Error,* 2nd ed. Santa Barbara, CA: Aegean Publishing, 1998.
  A collection of true stories about design-induced human errors describing how disasters are caused by incompatibilities between the design and humans. Many of the stories are health care–related.

Norman D.: *The Design of Everyday Things.* New York City: Basic Books, 1988.
  Uses everyday examples to demonstrate bad designs and the need for user-friendly designs. Examples are easy to relate to and use everyday language to explain human factors issues.

If you want to educate leadership about HFE in your health care organization

Bias R., Mayhew D.: *Cost Justifying Usability: An Update for the Internet Age,* 2nd ed. San Francisco: Morgan Kaufman, 2005.
  Offers specific techniques for quantifying the costs and benefits to build a convincing and successful business case for investing in usability engineering.

Schaffer E.: *Institutionalization of Usability: A Step-by-Step Guide.* Boston: Addison-Wesley, 2004.
  Intended for executives who are championing a change in product development processes throughout their organization. Offers practical guidance on how to get usability recognized and incorporated into an organization's values and culture.

If you want to get deeper

Carayon P.: *Handbook of Human Factors and Ergonomics in Health Care and Patient Safety.* Mahwah, NJ: Lawrence-Erlbaum, 2006.
  Provides several dozen chapters on the intersection of health care safety issues with the science of human factors. These range from how to use HFE to critique hospital computer systems to fatigue and repetitive stress injuries of nurses.

Dekker S.: *The Field Guide to Understanding Human Error.* Burlington, VT: Ashgate, 2006.
> Provides a theoretical structure for understanding the mechanisms behind human error and how HFE can help people understand and prevent errors.

Rubin J.J., Chisnell D.: *Handbook of Usability Testing: How to Plan, Design, and Conduct Effective Tests, 2nd ed.* Indianapolis: Wiley, 2008.
> Used by practitioners as a guide to usability testing, this book includes practical tips for integrating HFE activities into the software development process and provides templates and checklists to get you started.

Salvendy G.: *Handbook of Human Factors and Ergonomics,* 3rd ed. New York City: Wiley-Interscience, 2006.
> This 1,680-page handbook (encyclopedia) covers almost any conceivable aspect of HFE, from the mundane (anthropometrics and computers) to the exotic (joystick design for zero-G in spaceflight).

Weinger M., Wiklund M.E., Gardner-Bonneau D.: *Handbook of Human Factors in Medical Device Design.* Boca Raton, FL: CRC Press, 2010.
> This handbook includes HFE data and research that support evidence-based design and evaluation of medical devices and software. It has many similarities to the 2010 AAMI-HE75 guideline, which is likely to be cited and used by the U.S. Food and Drug Administration (FDA) and other policy groups.

Wickens C.D., et al.: *An Introduction to Human Factors Engineering,* 2nd ed. Upper Saddle River, NJ: Pearson Prentice Hall, 2004.
> Popular introductory human factors textbook. Covers the principles of human-system interaction and design, both cognitive and physical, along with examples to illustrate how they should be incorporated into the design of systems with which people interact.

If you want guidance for a design project

FDA Human Factors Program
Human factors guidance documents published by the FDA.
- ☐ Sawyer D.: *Do It By Design: An Introduction to Human Factors in Medical Devices.* http://www.fda.gov/MedicalDevices/DeviceRegulationandGuidance/GuidanceDocuments/ucm094957
- ☐ Callan J.R., Gwynne J.W.: *Human Factors Principles for Medical Device Labeling,* 1993. http://www.fda.gov/downloads/MedicalDevices/DeviceRegulationandGuidance/GuidanceDocuments/UCM095300.pdf
- ☐ *Medical Device Use-Safety: Incorporating Human Factors Engineering into Risk Management.* Jul. 18, 2000. http://www.fda.gov/downloads/MedicalDevices/DeviceRegulationandGuidance/GuidanceDocuments/ucm094461.pdf
- ☐ *Human Factors Points to Consider for IDE Devices,* 1998. http://www.fda.gov/MedicalDevices/default.htm

ANSI/AAMI HF74: 2001
American National Standards Institute/Association for the Advancement of Medical Instrumentation (ANSI/AAMI) 14971: *Application of Risk Management to Medical Devices.* Arlington, VA: Association for the Advancement of Medical Instrumentation, 2007.

Association for the Advancement of Medical Instrumentation: *Human Factors Design Process for Medical Devices.* Provides an overview of the HFE process and methods and techniques used in HFE processes. http://www.aami.org

ANSI/AAMI HE75:2009
AAMI: *Human Factors Engineering: Design of Medical Devices.* Arlington, VA: AAMI, 2009.
> This guideline provides more specific detail about how each aspect of a device and software should be designed—from minimal font size on a warning label to buttons on computer screens. It is likely to be cited by the FDA and other regulatory groups when evaluating adverse events.

Weinger M., Wiklund M.E., Gardner-Bonneau D.: *Handbook of Human Factors in Medical Device Design.* Boca Raton, FL: CRC Press,

APPENDIX
Human Factors Engineering Resources

2010 (*see* "If you want to go deeper" section).

MIL-STD-1472F. Department of Defense Military Standard: *Human Engineering Design Criteria for Military Systems, Equipment and Facilities*, 1999.
Detailed design criteria, principles and practices to be applied in the design of systems, equipment, and facilities.
http://www.hf.faa.gov/docs/508/docs/milstd14.pdf

NUREG 0700 (Revision 2). U.S. Nuclear Regulatory Commission's *Human-System Interface Design Review Guidelines*, 2002.
Detailed requirements on workstation design, alarms and warnings, computer-based procedure systems, information display requirements (e.g., icons and symbols, numeric data, color, indicators, cursors, scrolling), communication systems, and design of controls.
http://www.nrc.gov/reading-rm/doc-collections/nuregs/staff/sr0700/nureg700.pdf

If you want to browse the latest publications on HFE research or practical applications
Magazines
Interactions
Published by the Association for Computing Machinery (ACM) Special Interest Group on Computer-Human Interaction (SIGCHI), the magazine publishes articles on applied human-computer interaction for practitioners (users, developers, designers, managers, researchers, and purchasers).
http://www.acm.org/sigchi

Ergonomics in Design
A magazine on practical applications of human factors. Intended for practicing human factors engineers and ergonomists who are concerned with the usability of products, systems, and environments.
http://www.hfes.org/publications/ProductDetail.aspx?ProductID=36.

FDA's Patient Safety News
Broadcast and newsletter style summaries of adverse events involving medical devices—including many that cite human factors engineering design issues (e.g., Episode #78).
http://www.accessdata.fda.gov/scripts/cdrh/cfdocs/psn/index.cfm

Journals
Ergonomics
Official journal of the Ergonomics Society and the International Ergonomics Association. It is an international, multidisciplinary, refereed journal that publishes research on human factors and ergonomics.
http://www.ergonomics.org.uk

Human Factors
Official research journal of the Human Factors and Ergonomics Society. Publishes original papers on basic and applied research, quantitative and qualitative approaches to theory, evaluative reviews of the literature, and state-of-the-art reviews that cover all aspects of the human-system interface.
http://www.hfes.org/publications/ProductDetail.aspx?ProductID=1

International Journal of Human-Computer Interaction
International journal that publishes research on cognitive, social, health, and ergonomic aspects of work with computers.
http://www.elsevier.com/wps/find/journaldescription.cws_home/622846/description#description

IEEE Transactions on Systems, Man, and Cybernetics
This journal, published by the Institute of Electrical and Electronics Engineers, covers systems engineering, human factors and human machine systems, and cybernetics and computational intelligence.
http://www.ieeexplore.ieee.org

Human Computer Interaction (HCI)
An interdisciplinary journal, HCI publishes theoretical, empirical, and methodological articles on user psychology and computer

system design as it affects the user.
http://www.hci-journal.com

If you want to know more about specialty areas in HFE

Crandall B., Klein G., Hoffman R.R.: *Working Minds: A Practitioner's Guide to Cognitive Task Analysis.* Cambridge MA: MIT Press, 2006.

Dul J., Weerdmeester B.: *Ergonomics for Beginners: A Quick Reference Guide, 3rd ed.* Boca Raton, FL: CRC Press, 2008.

Fisk A.D., et al.: *Designing for Older Adults: Principles and Creative Human Factors Approaches.* Philadelphia : Taylor & Francis, 2004.

Goodrich M.A., Schultz A.C.: *Human Robot Interaction: A Survey.* Boston: Now Publishers, 2008.

Hancock P.A., et al.: *Human Factors in Simulation and Training.* Boca Raton, FL: CRC Press, 2008.

Hendrick H., Kleiner, K.: *Macroergonomics: Theory, Methods, and Applications.* Mahwah, NJ: Lawrence Erlbaum Associates, 2002.

Holtzblatt K., Wendell J.B.: *Rapid Contextual Design: A How-to Guide to Key Techniques for User-Centered Design.* San Francisco: Morgan Kaufmann, 2005.

Sears A., Jacko J.A.: *The Human-Computer Interaction Handbook: Fundamentals, Evolving Technologies and Emerging Applications,* 2nd ed. Boca Raton, FL: CRC Press, 2007.

Stanney K.M.: *Handbook of Virtual Environments: Design, Implementation, and Applications.* Mahwah, NJ: Lawrence Erlbaum Associates, 2002.

Stanton N.A., et al.: *Human Factors in the Design and Evaluation of Central Control Room Operations.* Boca Raton, FL: CRC Press, 2009.

Vu K.L., Proctor R.W.: *The Handbook of Human Factors and Web Design.* Boca Raton, FL: CRC Press, 2004.

Wogalter M., Frantz J.P.: *Handbook of Warnings.* London: Taylor & Francis, 2005.

If you want to browse for resources on the Internet

Association for Computing Machinery (ACM)'s Special Interest Group on Computer-Human Interaction

The main professional association in the United States for specialists in the HFE aspects of computer hardware and software. Many members come from computer science or engineering backgrounds and move into the HFE world.
http://www.sigchi.org

U.S. Department of Defense, Human Factors Engineering Data Compendium

Developed at the U.S. Air Force Research Laboratory, the compendium provides extensive data about capabilities such as language processing and visual acquisition of information.
http://www.dtic.mil/dticasd/edc/TOC/EDCTOC.html

ECRI Institute (formerly Emergency Care Research Institute)

This is one of the premier organizations in the United States that collects, analyzes, and reports recommendations to reduce medical device error, including specific emphases on HFE and usability attributes of devices.
http://www.ecri.org

Federal Aviation Administration (FAA) Web-based HFE Training

Designed by FAA human factors professionals for all the people in the FAA who build or buy devices and software (e.g., air-traffic control software).
http://www.hf.faa.gov/webtraining/Intro/Intro1.htm

Health Care Human Factors Group

University Health Network, Toronto, Ontario, Canada

This is a multidisciplinary group of clinicians and engineers who use HFE to assist the mission of the University Health Network hospitals, perform HFE analyses for industry, and conduct grant-supported HFE and health care research. They have a dedicated usability laboratory and provide HFE training (workshops and online) for stakeholders throughout the organization.
http://www.ehealthinnovation.org/?q=hhf

APPENDIX
Human Factors Engineering Resources

Human-Computer Interaction (HCI) Bibliography

Collection by a professor at The Ohio State University, which includes more than 1,500 Internet resources on HCI categorized and searchable in many ways.

http://www.hcibib.org/index.html

The Human Factors and Ergonomics Society

The main professional organization in the United States. Includes links to publications, regional professional groups, and academic programs in human factors engineering.

http://www.hfes.org

International Ergonomics Association

The main HFE professional organization for the international community.

http://www.iea.cc

Joint Commission International (JCI)

As the international division of Joint Commission Resources, JCI improves the safety of patient care through the provision of accreditation and certification services as well as through advisory and educational services aimed at helping organizations implement practical and sustainable solutions.

http://www.jcrinc.com/About-JCI

The Joint Commission

The predominant standard-setting and accrediting body in health care, the Joint Commission accredits and certifies more than 17,000 health care organizations and programs in the United States.

http://www.jointcommission.org/AboutUs

The Joint Commission Center for Transforming Healthcare

Launched in 2009, the Center works with leading health care organizations to identify and measure poor-quality and unsafe health care to develop and test targeted, long-lasting patient safety solutions. Many of these solutions, as applicable to such problems as hand hygiene and wrong-site surgery, are likely to involve consideration of human factors-related issues.

http://www.centerfortransforminghealthcare.org

Marquette University's Rehabilitation Engineering Research Center on Accessible Medical Instrumentation

Unique academic program that blends HFE with medical device design and evaluation, with the focus on rehabilitation and design for disabilities.

http://www.rerc-ami.org/ami

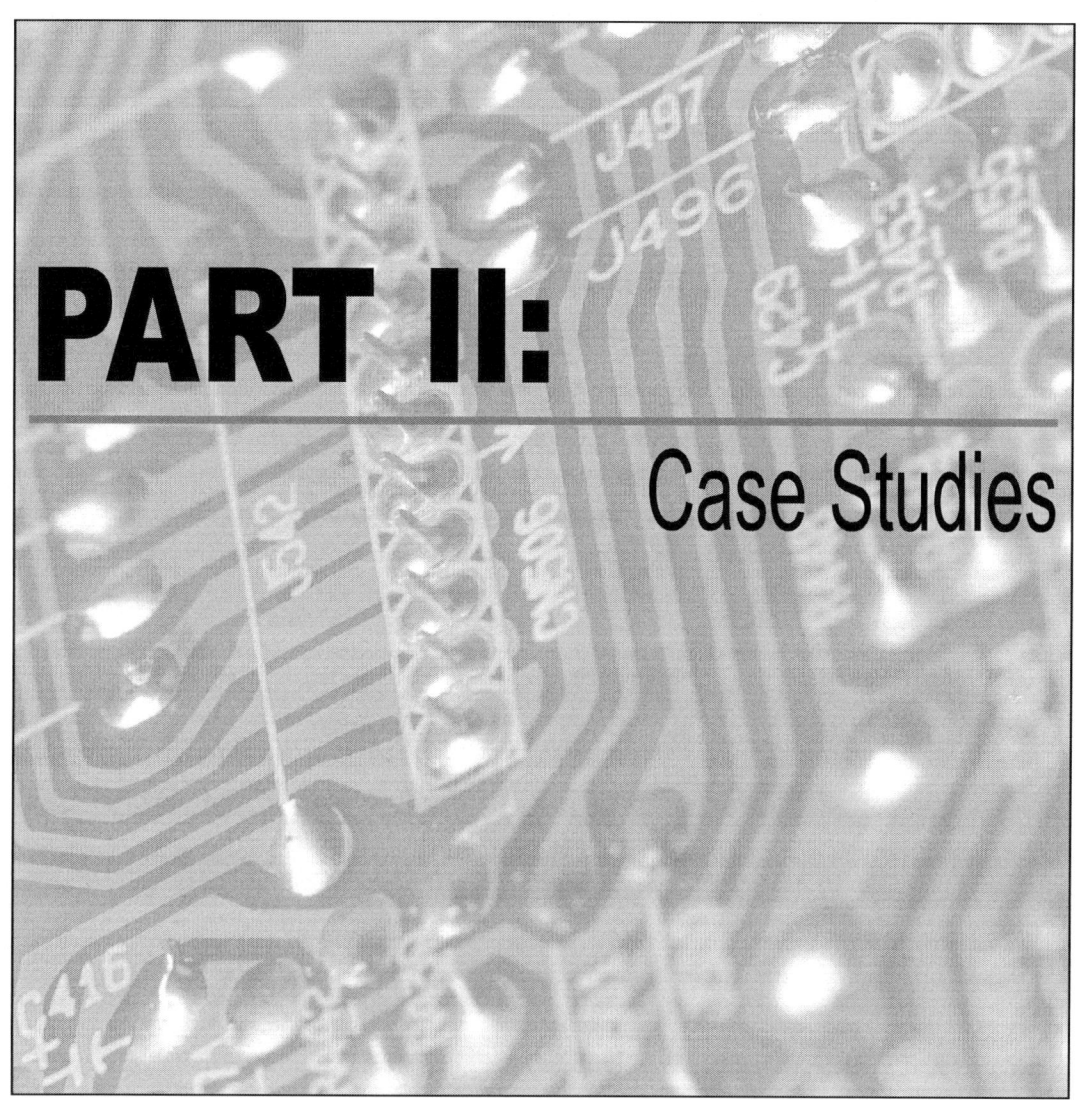

PART II:
Case Studies

Introduction

In Chapter 5, Sandra Coletta, a hospital senior executive who was already aware of the critical role of the human factors engineering (HFE) perspective in redesigning systems of care, reports how a fatal adverse event finally pushed HFE to the forefront of her organization's patient safety efforts. The hospital is building internal HFE expertise through executive training courses and by contracting with a local firm with expertise in HFE and health care improvement. A project to rethink and redesign the emergency department is in its early stages.

In Chapter 6, Edward Etchells charts his own evolution in appreciating, and then teaching others about, the role of HFE in understanding adverse events and improving patient safety. As the case studies show, training and involving practitioners in HFE can help promote interdisciplinary analysis of problems and implementation of solutions.

Peter Doyle relates in Chapter 7 that The Johns Hopkins Hospital hired him after its leadership become aware of HFE's applicability to health care. Although his position is in the biomedical engineering department, he collaborates with professionals in risk management, information technology, and a patient safety research group. In projects with clinicians and managers, he has helped with procurement, risk assessment of a proposed surgery work area, and training material redesign for emergency responders. On the basis of case studies of alarm management and supply processes for surgery-suite equipment, Dr. Doyle provides advice about how to fit HFE personnel into the hospital, including recognizing where HFE expertise will be particularly useful and noticed.

In Chapter 8, Laurie Wolf relates how her involvement as an HFE professional progressed from occupational health—employee safety—to patient safety. The way in which HFE can complement Lean Six Sigma is brought to life in an HFE training module for the Six Sigma black belt workshop. A subsequent case study—on improving equipment availability—illustrates how Lean Six Sigma and HFE can work together for good outcomes (wait times eliminated, lost equipment rate cut in half). Standout lessons learned from the HFE projects include the need to partner from the outset with (1) hospital departments that design and construct so that standardization and safety features are addressed and with (2) physicians or clinical leaders to determine how human factors interventions can best improve the work flow of care.

Chapter 9 follows the path of one human factors engineering expert, Yan Xiao, from his early interest in working in health care to his current role in patient safety research at a large academic medical center. This chapter provides insight into how an organization can "institutionalize" HFE as it integrates HFE expertise into patient safety research. The case study on information systems indicates the importance of outreach, education, and cross-training with information technology as it becomes an increasingly integral component of health care delivery.

Chapter 10 describes how the Institute for Safe Medication Practice Canada, whose mandate is to analyze medication incidents to make recommendations for medication system improvement, came to recognize the need for HFE as a core competency. In 2000, soon after the institute's creation, founding members with HFE experience and expertise pushed the organization to obtain training in HFE and team up with consultants. Learn how they used HFE to improve medication systems, as in, for example, designing a pre-hospital treatment kit for emergency medical services and conducting forensic usability testing after a fatal home-care chemotherapy mishap.

—John W. Gosbee, M.D., M.S.
Laura Lin Gosbee, M.A.Sc.

CHAPTER 5

How I Learned About Human Factors Engineering

Sandra Coletta

I can remember the moment when the light went on for me. I don't recall who was giving the presentation, where we were, or what the topic of the presentation was. I do know that it was around the time of the Institute of Medicine's *To Err Is Human* report.[1]

The speaker asked the audience whether they had ever arrived at work unable to recall the drive they had just made from home—which elicited a resounding "yes" from all the participants. She also asked whether any of us had ever left the house with our shoes on the wrong feet—of course not, we said, it would be uncomfortable. She then showed us a slide depicting animated moving vehicles, which were in a horrible traffic jam as the lights on the signal blinked in purple, blue, and orange.

From that day forward, I began to become more attuned to the role of human factors or human factors engineering (HFE) in everyday life. The cold-water faucet is always to the . . . ? I can't actually remember without going to the sink, but when I do my hand reaches to the right. I use a calculator frequently at work, only to wonder why I dialed the wrong number on the telephone so often. Then I realized that the layout of the numbers on the calculator was the reverse of the layout on my phone.

It was many years later when my boss at the time, an anesthesiologist, was recounting an event from early in her career. She was in the operating room (OR), providing anesthesia. During a crisis period in the case, she adjusted one of the dials on the anesthesia machine in the belief that the dial controlled one aspect of the gases, when, in fact—on this particular make and model—the dial served an entirely different function. That error almost cost the patient his life.

To me, the postscript to that story is what I found intriguing. I asked her what we needed to prevent the recurrence of that type of error. She smiled and said not to worry—the problem had been solved. At the urging of anesthesiologists, manufacturers standardized the placement of critical control dials on the machines. How obvious it seemed to me; after all, regardless of car make or model, the gas pedal is always to the right. On further research, I learned of the Anesthesia Patient Safety Foundation's other HFE–based efforts, including simulation training, alarms, and equipment innovation.[2] Why wasn't it expected that similar safety steps would be in place in all health care disciplines? What I realized is that health care, and hospitals in particular, were woefully unaware of the potential contribution of HFE. We had our improvement methodologies—for example, we studied Deming and Total Quality Management—and we knew how to brainstorm and do a root cause analysis (RCA) and flowchart, and so on. However, even when the RCA led to an equipment issue, it rarely focused on the interaction between the human and the machine. Most of these analyses resulted in communication and training issues. Off the staff went to the classroom to learn once again about how to implement the policy and procedure correctly. I realized that, unlike my "aha" moment, medicine did not offer training in HFE and that I hadn't learned how to consider the impact of human performance in complex systems.

The appropriate question one might ask at this point is, Why? We had entire staffs focused on quality assurance, which eventually evolved into quality improvement. We had inspections visits and accreditation visits and licensing requirements. Yet we seemed to leave out the essential component of the ability and limitations of the individual human charged with the task of providing high-quality and safe health care. Now, we did of course evaluate the individual, provide annual performance reviews, establish mandatory training, and assess competency. Yet, errors continue to happen. What were we missing?

In his recent book, *The Checklist Manifesto*, Atul Gawande, a surgeon and journalist, struggles with the same questions. In considering the difference between aviation and medicine, he identified a key difference in the expectations of professionals in these fields. In aviation, discipline in following prudent procedures and in working with others has become part of the culture. In medicine however, the physician's autonomy is a central principle. Dr. Gawande makes these observations in the context of the challenges faced in getting checklists used in the OR setting.[3] A surgeon colleague of mine, after observing a case in another institution, observed the same dynamic. In that setting, the nursing staff wore protective eyewear, but the surgeon did not. When asked why, the nurse explained that as employees they had to follow the policies and procedures of the hospital but they could only request the surgeons, who were not employed by the hospital, to do so. Each surgeon had the right to make his or her own decision as to using protective equipment.

If we believe that health care professionals are equipped to make the best decisions, have all the necessary knowledge, and process complex and sometimes conflicting information—and to do so for multiple patients simultaneously in chaotic environments—then we are sadly mistaken. The heroes of yesterday were those who took the risks, followed their intuition, and saved the day. The heroes today will be those who understand the system, plan for the worst, cite the knowledge of others, and recognize that their individual capabilities must be intertwined with the discipline to work with the system, the equipment, and the procedures that have been designed for safe outcomes.

LEARNING TO PUT HFE INTO PRACTICE

In 2006 I was the chief operating officer of The Miriam Hospital (Providence, Rhode Island). We had recruited a new chief of surgery, a pilot, who had a passion for patient safety. He and several of his associates had developed a course, "Lessons from the Flight Deck," which drew on the theory of crew resource management (CRM). The course cited some of the variables, such as communication and teamwork, situational awareness, fatigue, checklists, and briefings, that affected clinicians' performance—but had been missing from our approach to performance improvement. The course resulted in an increase in empowerment among staff and led to the decision to provide CRM training.[4,5]

CHAPTER 5
How I Learned About Human Factors Engineering

There was one aspect of CRM and other approaches to teamwork training, however, that created a nagging feeling in the back of my mind—CRM addressed only the human dimension of flight. Yet flying became safer not just because pilots learned how to work better with one another but because the manufacturers improved the mechanical, technical, and design features of aircraft. Similarly, in health care we needed to create a new approach to process improvement that used HFE to incorporate safety in the design of a process. As health care professionals, we were taking a successful effort—CRM—from another industry and layering it onto our broken infrastructure, and expecting it to achieve dramatic improvements in outcome. What we ended up with was a more open, aware, and collaborative workforce, but one that was still held back by the weight of processes that were decades old.

HOW A CONFLUENCE OF EVENTS PUSHED HFE TO THE FRONT BURNER

My fear that the lack of an HFE perspective in our approach to process improvement would be reflected in a medical error was realized on my last day at The Miriam Hospital, in September 2008. A surgeon operated on the wrong knee,[6] in spite of all the training and focus on patient safety, checklists, and teamwork, that we had instituted. From my new position as president of Kent Hospital, which was less than 10 miles from The Miriam Hospital, I watched with interest the steps that were then taken in response to the wrong-site surgery. In responding to requirements imposed by the state department of health, The Miriam Hospital engaged an HFE expert to provide education to the management team. In addition, to evaluate the process of ensuring surgery on the correct side for elective surgeries—starting with scheduling—it engaged a Rhode Island–based consulting firm, which specializes in HFE–centered design. I attended some of the sessions when the process of determining the correct surgery site was reviewed. As the many charts and work-flow analyses made clear, the number of times that information was transferred from one document to another, the number of unique individuals who touched a single document, and the multiple opportunities for error was staggering. I remember thinking that it was a miracle that wrong-site surgeries weren't even more frequent. However, I was encouraged to see that the design of the work process itself was being evaluated from a safety perspective.

During the summer of 2009, at Kent Hospital, in the case of one patient, a peripherally inserted central catheter (PICC) line was inserted in the wrong arm, and, in the case of another patient, the wrong hip was injected with dye for an imaging study. Both events occurred in the same department during a single week! The state department of health then came in to review these events and required us to conduct a detailed process review of the area where the errors occurred. In response, I met with the leadership of the same consulting firm that The Miriam Hospital had engaged to address wrong-site surgery to discuss what they could do to assist us. I told them that I was uncomfortable with the requirement that we focus on the area where the error occurred. Focusing on where the *last* error occurred represented a reactive approach that did nothing to protect us from the weaknesses inherent in our institution that had yet to be discovered. The message to the organization from this type of targeted intervention is that if something goes wrong, you will be visited by teams of experts who will fix you; so much for a teamwork model, open communication, and a nonpunitive culture. The consulting firm leadership agreed, confirming that although they could help make some improvements in a specific department, the reality of health care is that events reflect the

83

impact of a multitude of processes, which, to the novice, may seem unrelated. We talked about the need to begin at the beginning, back to the point where the patient first encounters the health care system and work our way through the flow of the patient's care, which ultimately would lead to the site where the errors occurred. Unfortunately, big projects require big budgets and lots of time. We had neither. The cost and disruption of retooling the entire way health care is delivered would be more than any single institution could manage. There was no way that our local hospital could take on such an endeavor. Or so I thought. At any rate, we hired the consulting firm.

Accelerating Toward HFE in Practice: The Michael J. Woods Institute

On December 1, 2009, Kent Hospital, midway through a significant, very public malpractice trial, announced that a settlement of the Michael Woods case had been reached. The settlement included the creation of the Michael J. Woods Institute, which would "focus on redesigning health care systems using a human-centered approach to improve clinical outcomes." The hospital committed to investing $1,250,000 in the next five years to redesign the care process, beginning in the emergency department (ED). The following excerpt is adapted from the official news release[7]:

> These efforts will be supported by a consulting firm with 25 years' experience in human factors–centered design, employing the expertise of researchers, engineers, social scientists, and medical professionals. This unique approach will create models of care that can be adopted by other hospitals across the country.
>
> "Human errors in the health care setting occur for a number of reasons, but at the root of many of them is poor communication. The weaknesses in the health care delivery system will only be eradicated when the human factor is considered in designing the solution," said Sandra Coletta. . . . "We know we're not perfect at Kent Hospital. Mistakes were made. We can do better. The Michael J. Woods Institute will help establish a leadership role in promoting patient safety and developing new ways to improve the patient experience and clinical outcomes."

The leadership of the institute will be guided by an oversight panel, including a Woods family representative, external experts, and hospital clinical leaders. A trained patient safety officer will coordinate the efforts on behalf of the institute on a daily basis. However, everyone involved made clear that this is much more than a new department or leadership role within the hospital.

The human-centered approach is founded in the belief that a hospital is a more dynamic environment than that expressed by any linear flow chart or regulated measures and metrics. Risks for system-safety breakdown exist in the nonlinear way that humans actually execute tasks—interacting with each other, their tools, and their environment. The work of the institute will be to identify risk-prone elements and implement innovative, risk-mitigating solutions.

Through a tragic event, we had found the way to do the impossible. We could take on the system, not just the single event.

The Case of Michael J. Woods

In 2006 Michael J. Woods arrived at the Kent Hospital ED complaining of acute onset of vomiting and severe pain in the region of his neck and throat, and died at the hospital of cardiac arrest several hours later. Michael was not placed on cardiac monitoring, even though it was ordered by the ED attending on the basis of the patient's condition and an abnormal electrocardiogram, during his time in the ED. After he was returned by stretcher from x-ray,

CHAPTER 5
How I Learned About Human Factors Engineering

he was placed in the hallway near the nurses' station because his treatment bay had been given to another patient. He suffered a myocardial infarction and became unresponsive and could not be resuscitated.

Michael, 49 years old, was active in our community; he had twice run for mayor of the city of Warwick, had three children, and he and his family had frequented Kent in the past. A malpractice case was brought by his only brother, James Woods, the actor, on behalf of the estate. The trial began in November 2009, and for its three-week duration, our hospital and the case of Michael J. Woods was front-page news in Rhode Island and elsewhere.

The evidence clearly indicated that the order for cardiac monitoring was not followed, as stated. The defense argued that the cardiac event was so significant that the monitoring would not have changed the outcome, while experts for the Woods family testified to the contrary. It was clear in my mind that we could have done better.

On November 30, 2009, I met James Woods for the first time and expressed our apologies for what had happened to his brother and acknowledged that we had not done everything that we should have. I told him that I had learned how the paper on which an order for cardiac monitoring is documented is placed in a folder on a counter, where a nurse is supposed to notice it and pick it up. Among other things I had learned, as I told Mr. Woods, were that (1) the handoff process when dinner breaks occur is not effective, (2) the physician's ability to access old records is limited, and (3) physicians are notified only if an abnormal x-ray result is received, not when the result is normal, even though the normal results increased the likelihood of a cardiac event in the differential diagnosis. I added that we have known for years that the process of health care is broken but that we have responded to each event with a Band-Aid, a new procedure, and more training but had not gone back to the beginning to design a safe process that incorporates HFE principles.

This case of Michael J. Woods and the institute has garnered attention from multiple fronts. The ability to settle the case, which was based on a willingness to acknowledge the error and take action to address it, has added a new perspective to malpractice litigation. Employees, physicians, board members, and community leaders have stepped forward to assist in any way they can. The multiple dimensions of people, process, and equipment must come together if we are to be successful. The key message to all those involved is that our work is not to make our existing health care system safer, it is to design safer health care systems.

HOW CAN YOU MOVE HFE TO THE FRONT BURNER?

I had been the CEO for less than a year when the opportunity to bring an HFE approach to our hospital arose. It was the first time in my career that I didn't have to try to sell my boss on the idea. I had tried to introduce the concept in previous roles but was forever greeted by blank stares, little understanding of the applicability to health care and a relatively soft return-on-investment (ROI) argument. When you venture into a new arena, the benefits are projected on the basis of the experience in other industries. It's hard to produce a hard and fast ROI under those circumstances.

I can readily understand the frustration that many people experience within their organizations when they can see the potential of HFE but don't have the leadership support to make it happen. That puts the responsibility squarely on the CEO's shoulders. In my case it was easy. I understood the basic HFE principles, wanted to give it a try, and was able to find a way to make it happen in a big way. But that won't be the case for most institutions. More likely, a problem will occur, the team will be assigned to investigate, and someone needs to speak up and suggest this approach. The CEO must either be the one to spark the thought or listen to the proposal when it is brought to him or her.

If you are a CEO reading this, kudos to you! If you are trying to persuade your CEO of the importance of HFE, then I suggest you share this book with him or her. If your CEO asks how much it would cost to use HFE, how many full-time equivalents would be needed, and so on, don't answer those questions. Instead, visit different areas of the hospital with the CEO, pointing out the everyday risks of patient harm and how HFE can be used to address them. Sometimes, when you know that an initiative will improve the quality and safety of care, you just have to undertake it. For example, The Miriam Hospital has earned the Magnet award (as recognition of excellence in nursing), and maintained it through three renewal cycles. Others would often ask if we had prepared a financial analysis or return on the investment, given the resources needed to meet the criteria. My response was that we didn't do one and that I never would. The return will be obvious in employee, physician, and patient satisfaction. If it isn't, you can always adjust course.

For me, redesigning our processes to reflect HFE will make Kent a better hospital. As CEO, it's my job to advance the organization that I am leading. What better way than to use a discipline that has been proven to enhance safety and introduce it to our environment.

Case Study: The ED Project

The first effort of the Michael J. Woods Institute is the redesign process in the Kent Hospital ED, which began in January 2010.

The research-and-discovery segment, whose key elements are shown in Sidebar 5-1 (page 87), took about four months. It began with the 10-week data-collection phase, during which the consultants spent considerable time in directly observing the ED, conducting extensive interviews and discussions with staff at all levels (patient input will occur in later phases), and analyzing downstream operations, such as radiology and laboratory, that affect ED operations. The consultants then conducted competitive assessment, mapping, and needs definition, which resulted in the identification of critical risks points. The critical risk points can be summarized into the broad categories of physical space reconfiguration, system protocols/policies, decision-making models, patient expectations, information tools/flow, and cultural foundation.

In the second segment of the redesign process—analysis and solution-building, risk- and severity-assessment tools will be applied to the identified risk points. Best-practice assessments from EDs and other industries will be introduced as Kent staff, along with the consultants, create scenario options. Critical to the success of this effort is the establishment of benchmark metrics to ensure that desired outcomes are achieved as solutions are tested. This phase will span a six-month time period, but we expect to begin the implementation of the solutions that can effectively improve the ED environment before all segments of the redesign are completed.

The scope of the redesign project is significant, involving a department employing 111 full-time equivalents, excluding physicians, that receives more than 60,000 patient visits a year. Oversight on a week-to-week basis has been managed by an executive committee comprised of the CEO, the chief nursing officer, the chief medical officer, and the senior vice president for

CHAPTER 5
How I Learned About Human Factors Engineering

Sidebar 5-1. Key Elements of the Research-and-Discovery Work Plan

- Human-centered ethnographic qualitative observations and contextual interviews of key stakeholders. Ethnography = "a descriptive account of social life and culture in a particular social system based on detailed observations of what people actually do."

- Movement of patient and patient information from first contact to disposition planning focusing on the following:
    - Triage process
    - Staffing, lab systems, information systems, documentation, bed shortages, etc.
    - Transfers of care
    - Prioritizing transfers, tests, and procedures
    - Patient identifiers
    - Communication tools (e.g., verbal, written, electronic)

- Institutional, departmental, and provider safety initiatives
    - Staff's and administration's understanding of safety initiatives currently in practice
    - Staff's and administration's understanding of near-miss reporting systems
    - Identification of unanticipated patient safety events
    - Safety initiatives that are planned for the future

- Organizational hierarchy across clinical and administrative departments
    - Reporting, staffing, and employment
    - Training and education

- Organizational aspirations
    - Vision for the future
    - Technologies and programs currently being planned for implementation in the near future

- Competitive landscape assessment to understand current industry "best-in-class" emergency departments as they relate to hospital systems safety

Source: Kent Hospital, Warwick, R.I. Used with permission.

---

human resources. In addition, a core team of nurses, physicians, and ancillary personnel has been assisting the consulting firm during the course of its work in periodic meetings, in which the team reviews progress against the work plan, reviews observations, and provides clarifications.

A local research team leader—a hospital-employed physician who is familiar with all aspects of the hospital, not just the ED—spends approximately 10 hours a week as the "go-to" person for the consulting firm, addressing problems as they arise and assisting with implementation of the work plan.

CONCLUSION

So many people have commented on the efforts at our hospital. The fact that we have acknowledged our weaknesses, owned up to errors made in the past, and recognized the continuing daily risk of harming our patients seems unusual to most observers. There is an expectation that hospitals and health care providers are unwilling to acknowledge that they are human and make mistakes. Perhaps it is because our mistakes often go unnoticed; for these mistakes there is no public tragedy, no 24-hour news reporter on site. We harm and sometimes kill patients one at a time. However, for the patient, family, and care providers themselves, the tragedy is no less real. We have worked on how to ensure that we hire the right people and continually monitor their performance. We have invested in information management systems and electronic medical records. We have state-of-the-art technology to ensure that we can diagnose and treat our patients.

But the mistakes still happen. I believe that HFE holds a key to the problem of medical errors, and I look forward to demonstrating the impact at our organization.

The author thanks John Gosbee for his guidance regarding this chapter; Mark Decof, J.D., for ensuring that the memory of Michael J. Woods was appropriately honored in the chapter; and the wonderful men and women who have stepped forward to serve on the Michael J. Woods Institute's oversight panel.

References

1. Institute of Medicine: *To Err Is Human: Building a Safer Health System.* Washington, DC: National Academy Press, 2000.
2. Hallinan J.T.: Once seen as risky, one group of doctors changes its ways. *Wall Street Journal,* Jun. 21, 2005. http://www.saynotocaps.org/newsarticles/once_seen_as_risky.htm (accessed May 3, 2010).
3. Gawande A.: *The Checklist Manifesto: How to Get Things Right.* New York City: Metropolitan Books, 2009.
4. Dunn E.J., et al.: Medical team training: Applying crew resource management in the Veterans Health Administration. *Jt Comm J Qual Patient Saf* 33:317–325, Jun. 2007.
5. Sax H.C., et al.: Can aviation-based team training elicit sustainable behavioral change? *Arch Surg* 144:1133–1137, Dec. 2009.
6. Freyer F.J.: Surgeon operates on wrong knee at Miriam Hospital. *The Providence Journal,* Sep. 20, 2008. http://www.projo.com/health/content/WRONG_AGAIN_09-20-08_A0BLGVG_v15.17c4c47.html (accessed Apr. 16, 2010).
7. Kent Hospital: *Press Release: From Loss Emerges Hope: New Michael J. Woods Institute at Kent Hospital to Focus on Redesigning Care Investment in the Redesign of Care Delivery System Announced in Conjunction with Settlement in Michael Woods Case,* Dec. 1, 2009 http://www.projo.com/news/2009/popups/kent-woods-release.htm (accessed Apr. 20, 2010).

CHAPTER 6

Human Factors Engineering in Action: Sunnybrook's Patient Safety Service

Edward Etchells, M.D., M.Sc.; Catherine O'Neill, R.N., B.Sc.N.; Jeremy I. Robson, Ph.D.; Richard Mraz, P.Eng; Julie Chan, B.A.Sc.; M.H.Sc.; Patti Cornish, B.Sc. Phm.

DEVELOPING AN INTEREST IN HUMAN FACTORS ENGINEERING

I first appreciated the relevance of human factors engineering (HFE) after 12 years of medical training and practice. During an incident investigation at a hospital, I met an HFE consultant, who pointed out error-provoking features of the health care environment that the rest of the "investigators" were not seeing. For one of the root causes of the incident—incorrect patient identification—the consultant observed that the hospital bradma cards (the colored plastic cards that state the patient's name, birth date, hospital file number, address, attending physician, and health insurance number, and which are a cornerstone of patient identification) were stored together on a rack. The cards were extremely difficult to read because of minimal contrast—the characters and the card were a similar color—creating a sea of indistinguishable plastic that promoted the likelihood of error. Worse still, the rack had slots labeled with room numbers (not patient names), yet the patient cards were often placed in the incorrect room number slot.

The incident also involved a late-night error in the programming of an intravenous infusion device. The consultant pointed out that a nurse would have had great difficulty programming the device in a darkened room at night because the keys were not backlit, so one could not see what was being pressed. Someone responded, "That's why nurses have flashlights," but the consultant was not daunted. He pointed out that the programming keys required significant pressure, but because the pump was on wheels, applying such pressure invariably caused the pump to roll away. He asked, "How can a nurse hold the flashlight in one hand, steady the pump with the other, then program the device correctly—with her third hand?" There was no good response. The system made no sense. HFE mattered. One of the nurses involved in this incident sent me a note thanking me for the supportive tone of the investigation. Although the note should really have been sent to the HFE consultant, it remains one of my most cherished possessions.

—*Edward Etchells*

HFE AND SUNNYBROOK'S PATIENT SAFETY SERVICE

Sunnybrook Health Sciences Centre (Sunny-

> **Sidebar 6-1. Cumulative Lessons Learned Regarding Human Factors Engineering**
>
> 1. HFE is highly salient with clinicians and hospital staff.
> 2. HFE is a connector—it promotes user-centered learning across disciplines, programs, and units.
> 3. Apply HFE principles when making decisions about new machines and software.
> 4. Large HFE projects require clinical and operational support.
> 5. HFE issues can easily be learned with low-fidelity simulations.
>
> **Source:** Sunnybrook Health Sciences Centre, Toronto. Used with permission.

brook) is a 1,200-bed academic hospital (700 acute care and 500 long term care beds) located in downtown Toronto. On an annual basis, it has 31,000 inpatient admissions for a total of 400,000 patient days and 10,000 inpatient surgeries; 42,000 emergency room visits; 6,000 outpatient surgeries; and 37,500 outpatient visits per year

In 2002 Sunnybrook established an innovations fund for local pilot programs. One of the funded programs was the error management unit, which was devoted to the identification, analysis, and reduction of harmful health care errors. In 2004, when the pilot project ended, a new Patient Safety Service was formally established within the Department of Quality, which was renamed the Department of Quality and Patient Safety. The error management unit's members—a physician director (0.4 full-time equivalent [FTE]; E.E.), a deputy physician director (0.1 FTE), a registered nurse (1 FTE; C.O.N.), and a pharmacist (0.8 FTE; P.C.), now constituted the Patient Safety Service. Our role was to develop and implement innovative patient safety programs for hospital staff. We quickly joined forces with the existing members of the quality department (including risk management) in creating and implementing patient safety projects.

In May 2002 one of us [E.E.] attended a Department of Veterans Affairs (VA) National Center for Patient Safety (NCPS) training course[1] and was inspired by the HFE presentations, as well as those provided on other occasions by Toronto-based presenters such as Kim Vicente, John Senders, and John Doyle. The cumulative lessons learned regarding HFE, which were spread to the other members of the Patient Safety Service, are listed in Sidebar 6-1 (above).

In spring 2002 the Patient Safety Specialists—the members of the Patient Safety Service—decided that disseminating and applying HFE principles were essential elements of a hospital safety program. We made this decision on the basis of the VA NCPS training session and two additional factors: (1) reliable design was recognized as a cornerstone of a safe hospital in an influential Canadian publication,[2] and (2) our clinical backgrounds (pharmacy, nursing, medicine) allowed us to appreciate the importance of HFE to safe clinical care.

In building Sunnybrook's HFE capacity, we had enthusiasm but a limited budget, so we chose to work with consultants on small projects rather than hire a full-time HFE expert. We did not have a clear view of the nature and amount of

CHAPTER 6
Human Factors Engineering in Action: Sunnybrook's Patient Safety Service

HFE work that needed to be done. We also wanted to develop our own HFE skill sets so we could be useful resources within the hospital. In all cases, the projects were short term (that is, less than one year), but we had a longer-term goal of building internal capacity and skill in HFE.

We found consultants almost entirely through word of mouth or through conferences. The HFE community in health care was very small, so there was no need to engage in detailed interviews or selection processes. In some cases, the consultants would refer to others if the project demanded. For example, some consultants were better oriented to large-scale usability testing, while others were more interested in the educational projects. In all cases, the consultants were hands-on participants in the projects because (1) they had content knowledge and were willing to share it; (2) their confidence and experience gave us confidence when it was our turn to provide a lecture or answer questions; and (3) they had practical operational experience with larger-scale projects, such as usability evaluation. We could not have done this on our own.

More recently, we have developed linkages to the University of Toronto engineering program. We wanted to link the operational activities in safety improvement to the academic mission of the hospital (education and research), which provides training for medical students and residents. We have had several student internship placements for focused projects and thesis projects for larger projects with a strong academic or scholarly aspect. Students bring a spirit of inquiry to the projects and allow us to make additional connections with engineering faculty.

Any member of the hospital staff can contact the Patient Safety Service for advice or consultation. We introduce ourselves at new staff orientation. The voluntary incident-reporting system is supervised by risk management, with whom we work closely.

Our educational offerings, which began with a half-day workshop in fall 2002, grew into a series of lunch-and-learn sessions, which in turn evolved into a formal HFE course, HF 101* (Case Study 1). As we developed confidence in our own skills, we began to apply these concepts to small safety projects in the hospital. For example, a small usability study on existing intravenous (IV) pumps led to the larger projects that informed hospital purchasing and implementation decisions—such as the smart infusion pump (Case Study 2), critical care information systems (Case Study 3), and computerized provider order entry (CPOE) systems projects (Case Study 4).

Case Study 1. Human Factors 101

We conducted the half-day workshop in fall 2002 as the first step in addressing our first objective—to raise awareness of human factors and its relevance to patient safety. The highlight of the workshop was watching our chief executive officer try to load a Pez dispenser with candy, a wonderful demonstration of how poor design can make it very difficult to complete an apparently simple task.

In the next step, we highlighted HFE in the 12-month series of "lunch-and learn" safety sessions. In one session, "Project Kodachrome," we gave each team a single-use camera and asked the teams to take snapshots of hazards and design problems on their units. These sessions led to the development of the Human Factors 101 course because of the participants' positive reactions to the material and desire for more knowledge.

---

* HFE and human factors are often considered synonymous (*see* Chapter 1).

The course, which we first offered in summer 2005, was based on work initially done in the neonatal intensive care unit (NICU) as part of the Vermont Oxford Network's NICQ project.[3] The topics for HF 101 included designing for safety, paper forms, labels and displays, alarms and warning devices, alertness and fatigue, procedures and task guidance (including reminders and checklists), usability, teamwork, and unit design and layout. We charged a nominal fee of $100 to cover printing costs, speaker costs, and refreshments.

During the next two years, we offered many internal Human Factors 101 courses and two external Human Factors 101 courses (provided at Sunnybrook for nonhospital staff) to a total of more than 260 participants—clinical staff from all health care professions, including nurses, nurse educators, pharmacists, speech language pathologists, physical therapists, occupational therapists, radiation therapists, and physicians. Laboratory staff, as well as staff from supply chain services, infection prevention and control, health data resources, and biomedical engineering, also attended, as did administrators (including managers, directors, vice presidents, and executive vice presidents). Clinical areas represented included emergency, neonatal intensive care, and internal medicine. Most of the courses received positive evaluations. The course on unit layout and design was not as well received, possibly because participants perceived no ability to change the layout and design of the units.

We found that HF 101 was valued by a broad range of hospital staff, including clinical and administrative staff from multiple disciplines and areas. The courses brought together members of the hospital who might otherwise never meet, let alone discuss safety issues, and sowed human factors concepts into the hospital. We stopped providing HF 101 in 2007 because we felt that we had reach a point of saturation among the interested staff. We continue to provide introductory presentations on human factors as part of nursing orientation. Some of the human factors material has been moved to the curriculum required for a universitywide certificate in quality and patient safety.

Early in the course, we used examples from everyday life, but the most consistent feedback to improve the course was to increase the number of health care examples for the small-group exercises that we developed for most of the modules. The participants also requested that the exercises be included in the take-home packages so that they could conduct them at their home units.

HF 101 (*see* Table 6-1, pages 94–95), was easily delivered in small groups in the hospital. Scheduling was a minor issue. We initially offered three half-day units, but we found that people did not attend all three sessions and that scheduling was too complex. We then shifted to a single-day course and compressed the material.

Our next step was to apply HFE knowledge to actual safety concerns within the hospital, with ongoing support from our expert consultants.

Case Study 2. HFE Evaluation of Smart Infusion Pumps

Our evaluation of smart infusion pumps was preceded by a preliminary simulation study that confirmed a role for HFE in developing hospital procedures and training programs. In spring 2005, reports received through voluntary incident-reporting system on incorrect dosing of high-risk IV infusions (heparin and insulin) were arriving regularly. The usual comment was that the nurse "did not program the pump correctly" or "programmed too high or too low a dose," but we suspected that there were important HFE issues to be explored. We created a study team that included representatives from nursing, biomedical engineering, and the simulation center to evaluate the usability of our existing IV infusion process.

We initiated the smart infusion pump project in 2008 after the hospital asked us for advice on the procurement of the then-new smart pumps, which have many capabilities and features that are intended to improve safety and reduce medications errors. For example, they have drug libraries that can be customized to meet the needs of clinical care areas and incorporate dose error reduction systems, which allow checking of the programmed dose against preset upper and lower limits to alert users to potential under- or overdosage of medication.

Our institution, having decided to replace our general infusion pump with a smart pump, issued a request-for-proposal, to which two vendors appropriately responded. The project team was composed of two Patient Safety Service members, program directors and managers, nurses, and biomedical engineers. The team members felt that a full-scale usability evaluation was warranted and advised involvement of outside consultants, which required the senior hospital leaders' agreement. Weighing the cost of the usability evaluation against the downstream costs of poor safety and efficiency, they decided that it made sense to make an informed judgment about the usability of a new device.

Usability Testing

Our objective was to conduct usability testing of smart pumps from the two separate vendors to determine ease of use and risk of error. Some 24 nurses, representing all the clinical care areas (intensive care, both adult and neonatal; cancer care; general ward) that would potentially use the pump, participated in formal usability evaluations of the smart pumps under consideration (Pump A and Pump B). Before each usability trial, participants attended a short training session (approximately one hour) with the pump's vendor. The testing occurred during two full days in our simulation laboratory, where human factors consultants observed the nurses as they programmed the pumps according to at least five separate clinical scenarios provided by clinical experts ("subject matter experts"). A sample scenario is provided in Sidebar 6-2 (page 96). During the observation, the human factors consultants completed a usability checklist. At the completion of the evaluation, all participants completed a questionnaire rating their experience with each pump.

The usability testing indicated that the participants encountered less difficulty selecting the correct clinical care area from the drug library with Pump A versus Pump B. Users reported that fewer steps were required to complete typical programming tasks with Pump A. Moreover, the participants made more errors when using Pump B than Pump A. The human factors consultants' evaluation determined that these errors with Pump B could be attributed to the following causes:
- Poor mapping between the physical system and display(s); there were several information sources available, resulting in confusion over which one should be prioritized.
- Ambiguous terminology on the display
- Nonintuitive interface design
- Unclear error messages
- Indistinguishable alarms

Pump A received significantly higher usability ratings than Pump B on a range of criteria. The usability score for Pump A was higher in all of the areas in which Pump B raised concern, with the exception of ease of use of the "Help" resources (*see* Table 6-2, page 97).

The results of the human factors evaluation

Table 6-1. Human Factors 101 Course Outline

Topic	Small-Group Exercise
Designing for Safety	
• Designing systems—we're all designers!	Identify a clinical hazard, including its source, its mechanism, and the nature of the harm.
• Safety improvement strategies and human factors	
Usability	
• Device and equipment usability principles and heuristics	Low-fidelity simulation of epinephrine pen administration (using training devices without needles or medication)
• Usability testing and evaluation	
• Identification of error potential and action	
Labels and Displays	
• Printed-label design factors	Analyze strengths and weaknesses of labels from SHSC and other hospitals. We showed photographs of labels and asked the group to apply the principles of label design.
• Device display characteristics, adjustment, positioning	Analyze devices from SHSC. We used our existing intravenous pumps and asked participants to attempt to program an infusion. If it was logistically difficult to have an actual device at the session, we showed pictures of the infusion pump keyboard and displayed messages instead.
Clinical Alarms and Warnings	
• Factors affecting the effectiveness of alarms	
• Auditory and visual principles for alarm information	
Procedures and Task Guidance	
• Procedure design and omission affordances	Analyze clinical procedure of drawing a routine blood test with a venipuncture, with focus on safety critical task step for removal of tourniquet.

(continued)

Table 6-1. Human Factors 101 Course Outline (continued)

Topic	Small-Group Exercise
Procedures and Task Guidance	
• Effective task support with checklists and reminders	Analyze clinical checklists in use at SHSC. We showed some checklists in current use at SHSC, such as a thoracentesis (chest fluid drainage) checklist. We applied the principles of checklist design to the checklists and generated lists of strengths, weaknesses, and improvements.
• Form design, affordance, and task mapping to minimize error	Analyze SHSC forms in current use (standard orders). We showed some forms from SHSC and from other hospitals. We applied the principles of forms design to the forms, and generated lists of strengths, weaknesses, and improvements.
Alertness	
• Qualitative effect of fatigue on performance and error potential • Sleep requirements and tools to self-assess alertness • Paper and online input (forms, flow sheets, order sets, etc.)	
Team Performance	
• Safety critical team performance factors • Team performance shaping factors	Use SBAR* to communicate a patient concern. We prepared an emergency clinical scenario. Participants simulated a clinical emergency communication regarding the scenario. Participants then analyzed the communication using principles of high-performing teamwork and structured communication.

SHSC, Sunnybrook Health Sciences Centre; SBAR, Situation-Background-Assessment-Recommendations. Small-group exercises were not provided for every topic.

*Leonard M., Graham S., Bonacum D.: The human factor: The critical importance of effective teamwork and communication in providing safe care. *Qual Saf Health Care* 20(13 suppl.):i85–i90, Oct. 2004.

Source: Sunnybrook Health Sciences Centre, Toronto. Used with permission.

> ### Sidebar 6-2. Sample Adult Intensive Care Unit Scenario: Norepinephrine Infusion
>
> This scenario is one of the five clinical scenarios provided by clinical experts for the usability-testing study.
>
> Your patient has been ordered a norepinephrine infusion to keep his mean arterial pressure (MAP) greater than 65 mm Hg. You mix the bag at double-strength (norepinephrine 8 mg in 250 mL of normal saline).
>
> - Start the infusion at 2 mcg/min.
> - The blood pressure (BP) remains low—increase the dose to 4 mcg/min.
> - There has been a precipitous drop in BP—the physician is at the bedside and asks you to increase the rate to 30 mcg/min.
>
> **Source:** Sunnybrook Health Sciences Centre, Toronto. Used with permission.

(usability checklist and user feedback) clearly favored Pump A over Pump B. The major attribute of Pump A that users preferred was its touch-screen technology, which provided high-quality, legible graphics with an intuitive sense of interaction. Pump A was preferred on the basis of ease of use and safety. The smart pump implementation committee also considered other factors such as information technology requirements, cost of pumps, cost of disposables such as infusion sets, the software's continuous quality improvement reporting system, and ease of future upgrades. The hospital's procurement team (composed of senior leaders), decided to move forward with Pump A.

The results of the project were also presented to the hospital's nursing committees and at our monthly hospitalwide safety rounds. These monthly rounds, which are an important element of the Patient Safety Service, are attended by an average of approximately 100 hospital staff and trainees from all disciplines, including medicine, nursing, pharmacy, risk management, quality, and patient safety.

This project illustrated the value of integrating usability testing into the decision-making process for the procurement of safety-critical, expensive medical equipment. It represented a successful integration of HFE data to a major hospital decision. There was already a major hospital commitment of time and resources to the procurement process. The incremental cost of the HFE evaluation ensured that the best decision for patients and clinical staff was made. The large scope of the study required a full-time commitment of two consultants, in addition to the two members of the Patient Safety Service (as noted), to complete the project. The 35 members of the smart pump implementation committee (including representation from all clinical disciplines) also made an extensive commitment.

The next case study provides another example of integrating HFE into procurement—this time for software—and of how the HF 101 principles were integrated into the organization.

Table 6-2. Scores on Usability Checklist for Pumps A and B

Criteria	Pump A	Pump B
System required mental calculations.	4.3	3.2
Error messages provided clear sense of severity.	5.9	3.8
Duration of info display was adequate.	5.3	3.1
Resuming work with the pump was easy.	6.1	3.7
"Help" resource was easy to understand.	3.0	4.0
Small errors required data deletion.	4.1	3.0
Error correction required minimal data input/deletion.	4.1	3.3
Participants felt in control of system.	5.0	3.9
Easy to understand which buttons control a given function.	5.5	3.3

1 = poor; 7 = excellent.

Source: Sunnybrook Health Sciences Centre, Toronto. Used with permission.

Case Study 3. Critical Care Information Systems

In winter 2008 Sunnybrook's critical care program wanted to purchase an electronic information system. The 15-member project team that was created was composed of program directors, patient care managers, advanced practice nurses, and staff nurses and physicians—as well as critical care program, information services, and Patient Safety Service staff. The project team's charge was to evaluate the usability of a critical care clinical information system (CC-CIS), which would be used by the five Level II and Level III ICU areas within the trauma, emergency, and critical care programs, as well as the NICU and the coronary care unit.

There are many considerations when choosing an information system, but the director of the critical care program's commitment that usability would be the major determinant for selecting the electronic information system represented evidence of the sustained effect of HF 101 and early consultations with HFE consultants.

Usability Testing

The usability testing required a major commitment from the clinical staff and the project team. One project manager and one patient safety specialist helped to coordinate the usability testing, including data collection and data management.

The project team made minor modifications to the usability checklist that was used for Case Study 2 (Table 6-2) to suit the specific aims of this project; for example, the word *pump* was changed to *computer* or *computer screen; buttons* was changed to *keyboard*. Usability testing and site visits were the most critical and informative phases in the evaluation process. Together, they provided opportunity for end users to interact and provide feedback on a live, working system. Some 32 clinical staff took part in the usability testing, during which they were asked to perform a series of routine tasks on each proposed vendor solution. Patient safety experts assessed their performance and conducted subsequent debrief interviews. Each participant was also

> ## Sidebar 6-3. Routine Clinical Task (Nursing Role) as Performed During Usability Testing
>
> The routine clinical task for nursing as performed during usability testing consisted of retrieval, entering, and changing of data. ABG, arterial blood gas; O_2, oxygen; BP, blood pressure; MAP, mean arterial pressure.
>
> *Retrieve Data*
> 1. Retrieve & review current medications.
> 2. Review nurses' note.
> 3. Retrieve & review 0820 hrs vital signs & ABG results.
> 4. Retrieve & review trend of O_2 stats & BP over past 24 hrs.
> 5. Retrieve and review morning x-ray.
>
> *Enter Data*
> Enter Levophed (norepinephrine bitartrate) order for 6 mcg/min to maintain MAP > 65. Document the insertion of a new triple lumen line.
>
> *Change Data*
> Change Levophed order to give a range of doses from 4-10 mcg/min.
>
> **Source:** Sunnybrook Health Sciences Centre, Toronto. Used with permission.

asked to complete a usability questionnaire examining ease of use, navigation, and system functionality. Metrics were then generated from the questionnaire for scenario completion, overall positive/negative feedback, and general usability. The routine clinical task for nursing, as performed during the usability testing, is shown in Sidebar 6-3 (above).

Selected results of the usability evaluation are provided in Table 6-3 (page 99), which are based on responses from the 27 of the 32 participants who responded.

A final score (out of 100) for each vendor was generated by summing the scores for each evaluation phase, multiplied by their preassigned weighting. The usability component weighed heavily in the overall score, along with the functional and technical capabilities of the system.

The final choice of vendor and system was the one with the highest overall score—but not the highest usability score, given the following reasons:

- The functional and technical issues were important parts of the final decision.
- The team realized that the usability scores for the chosen system were systematically lower because it was the *first* system tested, so users were less familiar with automated clinical systems in general. After reviewing all four systems, the users felt in retrospect that they had unfairly marked the chosen system low in usability. This highlights the importance of randomly assigning the order of testing or at least being aware of the potential for ordering effects when conducting usability trials.
- The final decision was also guided by on-site visits where usability in the clinical setting could be observed, and the usability of the

CHAPTER 6
Human Factors Engineering in Action: Sunnybrook's Patient Safety Service

Table 6-3. Representative Usability-Testing Results for Clinical Evaluators

Twenty-seven clinical users rated each system on a 5-point Likert Scale

Statement	Vendor A	Vendor B	Vendor C	Vendor D
The system was easy to use.	3.77	3.85	3.97	3.74
The screens were clear and easy to read.	3.52	4.19	3.93	3.91
It was easy to move from screen to screen.	3.77	4.19	4.07	4.07
It was easy to enter clinical information.	3.63	3.56	3.7	3.66
Overall, I am satisfied with this system.	3.63	3.77	3.73	4.05

Each statement was rated on a 5-point Likert Scale (1 = strongly disagree, 2 = disagree, 3 = neither agree nor disagree, 4 = agree, 5 = strongly agree).

Source: Sunnybrook Health Sciences Centre, Toronto. Used with permission.

chosen system was judged to be very good during the on-site visits.

The final case study relates to the usability, efficiency, and safety of a computerized medication order entry system.

Case Study 4. Usability of Computerized Provider Order Entry Systems

In March 2008 Sunnybrook was planning a pilot implementation of a vendor-provided CPOE system for medications. The Patient Safety Service and the CPOE implementation team wanted to conduct a usability evaluation of the proposed medications order entry system upgrade and use this evaluation to guide design decisions. The Master's of Health Science program at the University of Toronto recruited a human factors graduate student [J.C.] to take on this project for her thesis requirement.

First, we examined how closely Sunnybrook's CPOE interface design followed accepted human factors design principles of user-friendly interfaces. Three human factors graduate students, including the student leading the project, along with a clinician [E.E.], were shown how to log into the CPOE test order-set system and navigate to the order-entry screen before they performed their evaluations. Each participant was given the list of key usability parameters, such as visibility of system status, match between system and the real world, consistency and standards, and aesthetic and minimalist design.[1] Participants were asked to explore the Sunnybrook CPOE system interfaces and document observations related to these usability parameters. Participants completed their evaluations independently, and were instructed to continue compiling feedback until all relevant interfaces were explored.

Next, on the basis of the data obtained from the first step, the graduate student designed a user-centered design interface for comparative purposes. Key features of the format included the preservation of the current provider ordering model; the ability to review all orders in one screen; the use of only checkboxes, drop-down lists, and free-text fields for user inputs; and a more simple and aesthetically pleasing interface. The user-centered design performs basic-error checking on user inputs. Specifically, all mandatory fields (for example, physician's name and pager number) must contain information before the order is accepted. In addition, items that become activated because of a user selection must also be acted on before submission is allowed. For example, if the checkbox for "Team" under "Admitting Team and Diagnosis" is selected, the drop-down list next to "Team" will activate, and the user must then make a selection from this list or deactivate the list (by deselecting the checkbox) before the user-centered design will allow the user to submit the order set.

Usability Testing

We conducted usability testing with 27 clinical volunteers using a test system (no orders were submitted for real patients). The study of CPOE test platforms with order-set functionality was conducted in a training room at the Sunnybrook information services department. A randomized trial design was used for the study, so all participants were assigned to each of the three formats—paper, the user-centered design, and Sunnybrook CPOE—in random order to minimize the potential for ordering effects. The computers in the training room were set up with 23-inch (58.4-centimeter) monitors and the necessary software applications (Sunnybrook CPOE order-set system and commercially available usability software). The software provides the capability to capture data such as screen video, screen text, audio, mouse clicks, Web-page changes, window events, observer input, keyboard activity, and survey responses. For the usability study, the software recorded the screen activity of the participant's computer, survey responses, and observer input from the observer computer.

Main Measures

Participants were asked to enter admission and medication order sets using the three formats—paper, Sunnybrook CPOE, and user-centered design. From the collected data, the three order set modalities were evaluated and compared on the basis of their efficiency, safety, and usability, as defined below:

- *Efficiency* was defined as the time to complete the ordering tasks, which was calculated by the usability software, using task-start and end-point markers placed by the experimenter during each session. Task-start points were marked when participants, selected the order set folder in either the Sunnybrook CPOE or user-centered design systems or put their pen to the paper order set forms. Task-end points were marked when the participant pressed the "submit" button in either electronic system or when he or she handed the paper form to the experimenter.
- *Safety* was defined as the number, type, and potential severity of errors in the submitted orders.
- *Usability* was defined as the number of times the participant requested assistance and by responses to posttask surveys. User satisfaction in terms of usefulness of the software, satisfaction with the functions/features, and the perception that the software supports the tasks as needed by the user were rated after the test session on a 5-point Likert scale in a poststudy questionnaire. Other measures, such as the user's perceived levels of frustration, confidence, and satisfaction with each task were determined through a posttask survey (all surveys were specifically developed for this study). Other data sources included observations made by the experimenter, feedback from the user during testing (participants' thinking aloud), and feedback from the user on completion of testing.

Results

The quantitative analysis of this study is ongoing. However, concerns identified by clinicians during the testing caused us to defer implemen-

Table 6-4. Selected Design Problems and Solutions from the Computer Provider Order Entry (CPOE) Usability Evaluation

Design Problem	Design Solutions
Users cannot easily review orders before submitting them.	Provide an ordering-summary option before submission so providers can easily review important information.
Users are distracted by large amount of drug information (for example, drug formulations, pharmacy dispensing system codes) that is not relevant to the ordering provider.	Hide information that is irrelevant to the user. Give user the option to review such information.
Users are confused because drug information is not presented in typical, logical order, but is instead presented in the following order: name, frequency, route, dose, unit of measure. Dose and unit of measure information is at bottom of screen and is difficult to find.	Display drug information in a typical, logical, organized manner: drug name, dose, unit of measure, route, frequency.
The drop-down lists for frequency and dose are long and confusing. Most options would rarely or never be chosen.	Reduce the length of drop-down lists, including only the most frequently used options rather than all possible options. Give users the option of choosing "other."

The important lesson from this case study was that our senior leaders supported the usability evaluation and supported the CPOE implementation team's decision to defer implementation on the basis of the usability concerns. This sent a strong message to hospital clinicians that usability is a prime consideration in software design and implementation.

Source: Sunnybrook Health Sciences Centre, Toronto. Used with permission.

tation until we could design solutions to address the fundamental design issues (*see* Table 6-4, above); all the solutions are now being pursued.

SUMMARY

The Patient Safety Service's experience with HFE at Sunnybrook has been uniformly positive. Health care professionals have generally recognized the value of HFE concepts and applications in theory; buy-in comes with experience, as in Case Study 4. HFE methods, such as simulation and participant observation in usability testing, have been easy to integrate into clinical settings. We recognize that larger-scale evaluations (Case Studies 2–4) particularly require senior leaders' commitment to make the necessary resources available. Such a commitment must reflect an understanding of the importance of having the HFE–informed information to make a wise procurement decision, even if the benefits of that decision may be difficult to quantify, particularly in the short term. By contrast, evaluations of existing hardware, which we undertook, for example, in preliminary simulation study to evaluate the usability of our existing IV infusion process, as explained in Case Study 2, yield fewer actionable effective recommendations. Such projects often provide the evidence base for future capital/resources investment and for recommendations for educational and training programs.

Through a simulation study, we identified several usability problems related to the infusion-device design,[4] which we used to modify our training procedures on how to use the pump. The findings were also included in our nursing orientation seminars so newly hired nurses could appreciate the role of HFE in the hospital's Patient Safety Service. Although there were no budgeted resources to replace the IV pumps, which had already been purchased, this endeavor illustrated the value of providing usability data when making future procurement decisions, as outlined in Case Studies 2 and 3. Integrating usability testing into the procurement process allows us to make the best decision regarding the procurement and implementation of new technology. Usability testing also helps us to proactively identify safety concerns that will require additional safeguards.

HFE remains integral to Sunnybrook's patient safety efforts, as represented, for example, in the following areas:

- Principles of forms and order-set design regularly cited at the forms committee and health records committee meetings.
- Large procurements are now informed by usability evaluation.
- User-centered design of human-computer interfaces is a primary consideration for any new health care applications that we develop or purchase.
- To advance teamwork, the simulation center is used for training, and an educational program focused on teamwork has been developed.

The authors acknowledge Dr. Donald Redelmeier, who conceived the idea of the Error Management Unit and has served as Deputy Director, Patient Safety Service, since 2004. The authors express their gratitude to the HFE consultants who have inspired and guided us: James Handyside (Improvision Healthcare), John Gosbee and Laura Lin Gosbee (Red Forest Consulting), and Lora Bruyn Martin (HumanSystems). The authors also acknowledge the contributions to the work described in this chapter made by Guna Budrevics, Charlene Boston, Sandra Knowles, Beth Johnson, Cynthia Bailey, Wendy Gilmour, and Debra Carew.

References

1. Department of Veterans Affairs (VA) National Center for Patient Safety training course: May 2002, Las Vegas.
2. Baker G.R., Norton P.: Making patients safer! Reducing error in Canadian healthcare. *Healthc Pap* 2(1):10–31, 2001.
3. Handyside J., Suresh G.: Systematic application of human factors and ergonomics in the neonatal ICU. Paper presented at the Healthcare Systems Ergonomics and Patient Safety conference. Jun. 25, 2008, Strasbourg, France.
4. Zhang J., et al.: Using usability heuristics to evaluate patient safety of medical devices. *J Biomed Inform* 36:23–30, Feb.–Apr. 2003.

CHAPTER 7

Human Factors Engineering at The Johns Hopkins Hospital

Peter A. Doyle, Ph.D.

COMING TO JOHNS HOPKINS AS A HUMAN FACTORS ENGINEER

It is fitting that The Johns Hopkins Hospital (JHH; Baltimore) would have a human factors engineer on staff, given that the late Alphonse Chapanis, professor emeritus at The Johns Hopkins University, is considered one of the founders of the human factors profession.[1] However, it was in 2006 that John Gosbee, who was consulting for JHH at the time, persuaded the vice president of medical affairs of the value that human factors professionals could add to efforts to control factors that affect patient safety.

How do you hire and place a human factors engineering (HFE) professional in the hospital structure? A review of patient safety events indicated that the hospital would benefit from a human factors engineer who was attentive to issues of medical device design and selection as well as process design. One likely place for such a person would be the clinical engineering department, where he or she would have access to the engineering expertise and operational know-how of clinical and biomedical engineers. And that, fortunately, is where JHH placed its first human factors engineer, affording an opportunity for the person to learn the ins-and-outs of medical device use while also accepting assignments with clinical professionals on process issues.

Although the hospital sought a junior-level person, my experience as a human factors engineer in nuclear power and defense industries, as well as in the fields of human-computer interaction and telecommunications, was helpful in making a successful argument for the hiring of a more senior applicant.

ROLE OF HFE AT THE JOHNS HOPKINS HOSPITAL

JHH, a teaching hospital with 1,085 licensed beds, offers comprehensive medical and surgical services to patients from all reaches of the world. As the premier clinical center of an integrated health system that includes three other hospitals, JHH manages more than 97,000 inpatient admissions and 99,000 surgeries annually and provides extensive outpatient services.

With due regard for issues pertaining to its patients' well-being, the hospital has established various departmental and administrative offices, programs, policies, committees, and working groups to ensure the safety of patients in its care, conduct research on patient safety, and educate its own and other caregivers.

Principal among these are the board of trustees quality improvement (QI) committee, the QI council, operations integration administration, the quality and safety research group, and the risk management and patient safety committees.

Many, perhaps even most, human factors "engineers" are not formally trained in the specific industry in which they work. In my experience, many received their training in the social sciences (for example, in applied experimental psychology). Although such persons bring unique knowledge and skills to the table, they must learn the industry-specific subject matter. Use of HFE methods such as function analysis (identifying the functions required to complete a process) and task analysis (analyzing and decomposing the specific actions required) are of great assistance in speeding up and advancing the learning curve. These two analytic tools are valuable aids in identifying performance-shaping factors (PSFs)—factors or conditions found in the systems domains of knowledge, skills, and abilities (KSAs) and environment, tools, procedures, and other conditions that shape system performance.

As the human factors engineer at JHH, I report organizationally to the director of clinical engineering, who assigns a varied range of projects within the hospital setting. Other projects may be initiated by an e-mail, a phone call, or an impromptu meeting with clinicians in a hallway. Inquiries can be simple requests that result in a short answer or a detailed study. One simple request addressed the issue of possible errors using a patient-controlled analgesia pump, which were attributed to improper use of color coding for individuals with color-vision deficiencies. After quick review, the color coding was reinforced with text identifying the drug, so dual media were provided for conveying the information. Also, red was not used so there was no problem for the more common red/green deficiencies.

The clinical engineering department provides my funding, and the scope of my work is not limited by grants or specific contracts. Therefore I have the flexibility to apply my skills both proactively by investigating the potential for harm and reactively by addressing safety issues as they arise.

Recent projects have included the following:
- Safety evaluations of new and existing devices, workplaces, work spaces, and tools—such as software-based tools (for example, an electronic medication administration record) and alarm management (Case Study 1, page 105)
- Identifying and evaluating risks—such as evaluating the use of tubing products in view of possible misconnections
- Processes analyses—such as evaluating measures to control packaging, labeling, and processing of biopsy materials for accurate biopsy identification
- Simulation of emergency-response events for purposes of both discovery and education—such as simulations of delivery and use of emergency airway tools.

Projects range from short term (such as evaluation of operating room [OR] fracture-table control systems) to long term (such as a customized nurse call-system). I have addressed product safety issues with vendors and U.S. Food and Drug Administration (FDA) representatives, analyzed device maintenance and operations issues with biomedical technicians, and helped resolve work-space issues for anesthetists. Determining the requirements for information displays in ORs is an example of a needs analysis conducted with clinical engineering personnel.

No matter the project, HFE depends on collaboration with clinical engineers, clinicians, and administrators in the effort to determine the applicable performance issues. For example, nurses and clinical engineers provided their expertise in a hazard analysis of an infusion pump design, and nurses, along with procurement and product specialists, were instrumental in a tubing misconnection study. At an anesthesiologist's invitation, working with physicians, nurses, equipment specialists, and others, I participated in airway-cart and unannounced emergency-drill simulations to evaluate all aspects of emergency-airway services. We evaluated the emergency-cart delivery process and communication, teamwork, and equipment issues—which later enabled me to contribute to the development of training materials for emergency-airway procedures.

As a human factors engineer, I also interact with our risk management office, not only to assist in root cause analyses but also to learn from their risk and clinical perspectives. Collaboration with risk management promotes learning about precursors to adverse events, which in turn facilitates improvement of hazard analysis skills. On the other hand, examining issues with a human factors engineer enables risk managers to learn new ways to mitigate risk. For example, when examining controls to prevent burns from an infrared light used for skin treatments, I was able to educate a risk manager how to assess the adequacy of the warning decal design, including its placement in accordance with standards established by the American National Standards Institute.[2]

The following case study describing a fault tree analysis (FTA) undertaken as part of The Johns Hopkins Hospital alarm management task force shows the role of HFE in a more detailed study.

Case Study 1. Use of Fault Tree Analysis for Alarm Management
Background
One vexing problem facing many hospitals is the control and management of the many alarms used to alert clinicians to declining patient conditions. The outlook for improving alarm management looks challenging, given the increasing numbers of the following:
- Devices and systems with clinical alarms
- New features within devices that have alarms
- Ways to notify clinicians of alarms
- Beds in clinical units
- Patients requiring alarm monitoring

Moreover, the high percentage of false or clinically insignificant alarms further complicates the challenge of enabling reliable alarm detection and proper response. ECRI Institute recently placed "alarms on patient monitoring devices" as the number two health technology hazard (following cross-contamination from flexible endoscopes), accounting for 2% of the nearly 2,200 medical device problems reported between 2000 and 2006.[3]

Method
In 2007, as a human factors engineer, I was invited to join an alarm management task force that included nursing, clinical engineering, information technology, and vendor representatives. We decided to perform a FTA to identify possible causes of failures to respond to auditory physiologic alarms requiring action at the bedside (such as crisis alarms or "leads off") or failure to respond in a timely manner.

A Failure Mode and Effects Analysis (FMEA) or hazard or risk analysis is an inductive process that begins with a condition or event and ultimately determines its effect on the system. In contrast, in an FTA, we suppose a system failure and through a deductive process determine what events could contribute to that failure.[4] As

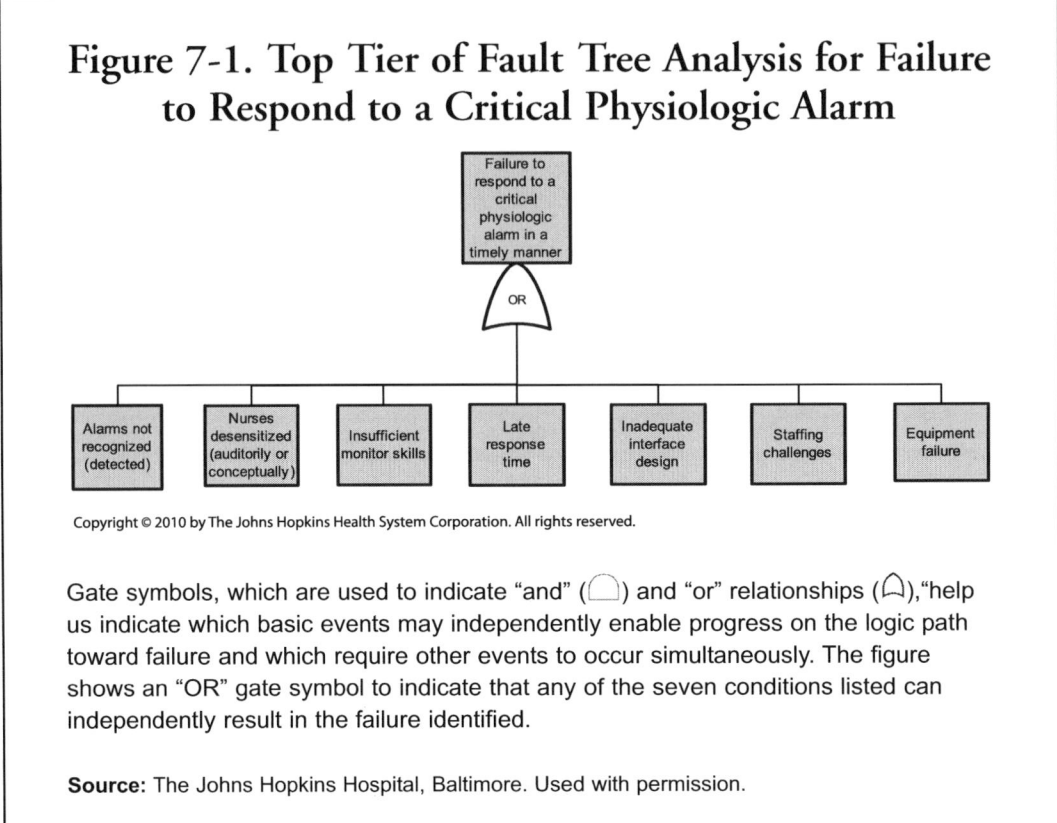

Figure 7-1. Top Tier of Fault Tree Analysis for Failure to Respond to a Critical Physiologic Alarm

Gate symbols, which are used to indicate "and" (⌂) and "or" relationships (⌂),"help us indicate which basic events may independently enable progress on the logic path toward failure and which require other events to occur simultaneously. The figure shows an "OR" gate symbol to indicate that any of the seven conditions listed can independently result in the failure identified.

Source: The Johns Hopkins Hospital, Baltimore. Used with permission.

such, an FTA is one of many analytical techniques that are useful in a root cause analysis (RCA) activity. The contributions to failure are documented in a tree-like figure showing relationships among basic events (initiating events), intermediate events, and the top event (failure). The figure should show the "parallel and sequential combination of faults that will result in the occurrence of the predefined undesirable event."[4]

In the fault trees shown in Figure 7-1 (above) and Figure 7-2 (page 107), the top event is "Failure to respond to a critical auditory physiologic alarm in a timely manner." In the case depicted, as a human factors engineer, I helped the alarm management task force define the top and contributing events to failures. A well-defined top event is important in that it con-

fines our analysis to the specific area of interest. Gate symbols help us indicate which basic events may independently enable progress on the logic path toward failure and which require other events to occur simultaneously. Of course, after the events are identified as risks to patient safety, analysts can proceed with identifying preventive measures.

Resulting Recommendations

For each of the intermediate events identified in boxes in Figure 7-1, the team identified a number of subordinate intermediate events and associated initiating events (circles) in Figure 7-2. Some of the corrective actions for the "Alarms not recognized (detected)" event are shown in Table 7-1 (page 108), while Table 7-2 (page 109) shows corrective actions for "Nurses desensitized"—referring to an effect of *alarm*

CHAPTER 7
Human Factors Engineering at The Johns Hopkins Hospital

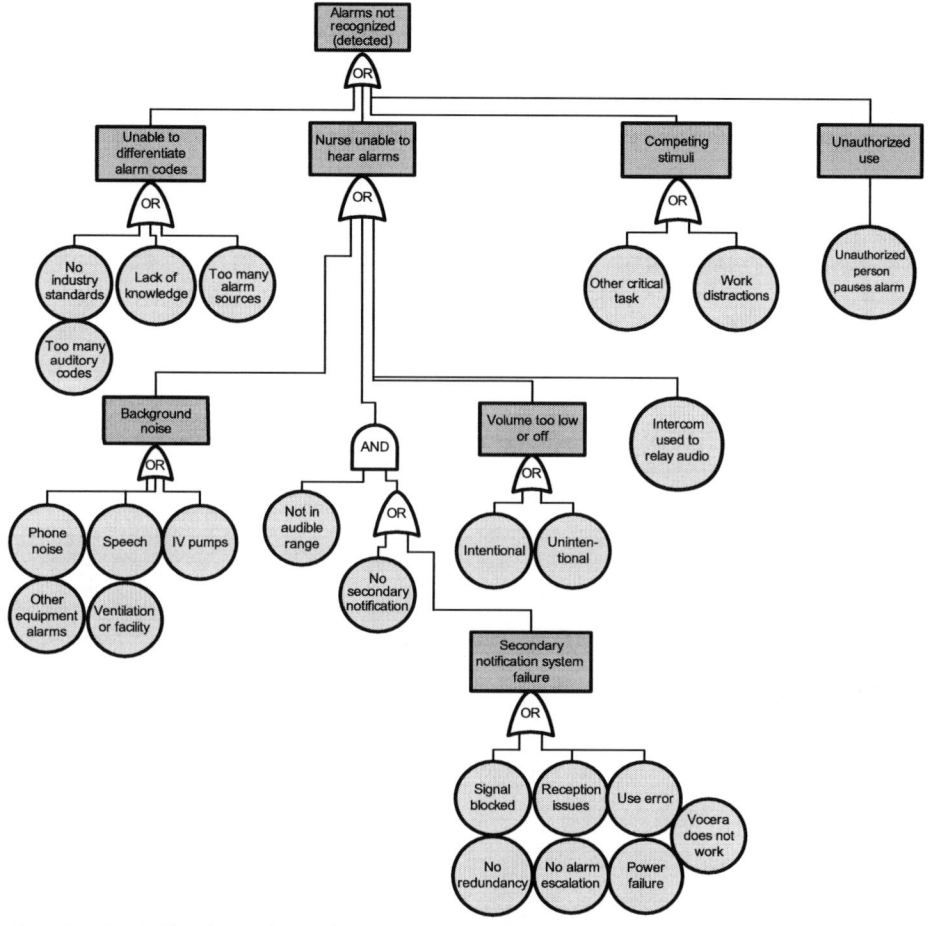

Figure 7-2. Fault Tree Analysis of Initiating Events for the Intermediate Event "Alarms Not Recognized"

Copyright © 2010 by The Johns Hopkins Health System Corporation. All rights reserved.

Initiating events (in circles) may independently, or in concert with other initiating events, result in intermediate events (boxes), ultimately resulting in a failure (top event).

Source: The Johns Hopkins Hospital, Baltimore. Used with permission.

fatigue. Table 7-3 (page 109) shows the corrective actions taken for "Inadequate interface design."

Status and Outcome of Corrective Actions
Evaluations of the candidate secondary-alarm notification systems continue. A program is now in place to evaluate one-way and two-way pagers, and an assessment of paging-system escalation features is also in progress (Table 7-1). Finally, the infrastructure of one unit has been upgraded for evaluation of wireless phones as a means of secondary notification.

> ### Table 7-1. Corrective Actions for "Alarm Not Recognized (Detected)"
>
> **Event:** Nurses unable to hear alarms
> **Corrective actions**
> a. Conducted a survey of other hospitals to determine types of alarm notification systems used
> b. Assessed various alarm notification systems available
> c. Identified candidate secondary alarm notification systems
> d. Identified and implemented upgrades to software that enables views of other monitors from one bedside
> e. Revised policy governing alarm-volume control
> f. Added speakers in select areas as supplemental sources for alarm audio
> g. Planned project to evaluate clinical alarms in two hospital towers under construction from a systems standpoint
>
> **Event:** Too many alarm sources
> **Corrective actions**
> a. Compiled alarm parameter thresholds for various clinical areas
> b. Identified most frequent alarms
> c. Assessed the inventory of alarms in the clinical environment and the need/value
> d. Implemented changes to alarm thresholds using data obtained and in consultation with the vendor's clinical specialist
> e. Implemented an alarm watch (dedicated nurse to watch a central display of all patients) for better recognition of alarms, tracking patient status and notifying floor nurses of patient conditions
>
> **Event:** Not in audible range and/or secondary notification system failure
> **Corrective actions**
> a. Developed training and procedure to replace/recharge batteries on a scheduled basis
> b. Trained staff not to use pagers as primary system
> c. Developed procedures and training to instruct users to stay within audible range of alarms
>
> **Source:** The John Hopkins Hospital, Baltimore. Used with permission.

By implementing these and other solutions not provided in Tables 7-1 to 7-3, the task force helped reduce the number of alarms on the cardiac care unit from 500 plus per patient day to approximately 250 within the course of one year.

The next case study entailed an analysis of the PSFs, which, again, affect performance of the system as a whole.

Case Study 2. Equipment Supply
Background
The perioperative environment can be a very busy, sometimes even hectic, place. All hospitals face the challenges of ensuring that proper OR

CHAPTER 7
Human Factors Engineering at The Johns Hopkins Hospital

Table 7-2. Corrective Actions for Intermediate Events for "Nurses Desensitized"

Event: Too many alarms
Corrective actions
Implemented a standards-of-care protocol that instructs clinicians to limit alarm monitoring to actionable alarms

Event: High false-positive rate
Corrective actions
Implemented training and a standards-of-care protocol that instructs clinicians in the proper techniques to reduce false alarms

Event: Failure to customize alarms
Corrective actions
Implemented training and bedside protocol changes that instruct authorized prescriber to order parameter thresholds and nurse to ensure that appropriate alarm limits and levels are set within two hours of admission

Source: The John Hopkins Hospital, Baltimore. Used with permission.

Table 7-3. Intermediate Event: Inadequate Interface Design

Event: Use of silence button for multiple purposes (to silence, to pause during alarm mode, to reactivate the alarm, to pause in the absence of an alarm)
Corrective actions
a. Developed and implemented training regarding proficiency of the silence button features
b. Conducted proficiency checks
c. Developed plan to evaluate human factors design considerations in future equipment purchasing

Source: The John Hopkins Hospital, Baltimore. Used with permission.

---

equipment is in place and ready for new cases and ensuring that urgently needed equipment is delivered quickly and in ready condition. In response to a request from an anesthesiologist to improve the likelihood that equipment is delivered on time and ready for use, I conducted a human factors analysis of PSFs. I analyzed various aspects of the system, investigating "non–person centric" factors such as the work environment, tools and procedures, as well as the "person-centric" factors of KSAs and motivation, communication, and teamwork.

> **Sidebar 7-1. Objectives for the Equipment Supply Project**
>
> 1. Achieve proper equipment availability by ensuring that equipment specialist personnel can do the following:
>   - Understand their roles for specific equipment in view of other personnel (e.g. critical care techs and nurses)
>   - Know where equipment is
>   - Know its condition at all times
>   - Maintain correct inventory in emergency carts
>   - Respond quickly to redeploy equipment
>   - Improve technical competency
>   - Prioritize tasks accurately
> 2. Ensure that the "system" supports execution of assigned tasks.
> 3. Establish a means to audit performance.
>
> **Source:** The John Hopkins Hospital, Baltimore. Used with permission.

The equipment specialist (ES) technicians at JHH report to an equipment manager, who helps establish their work duties, coordinates their efforts within and across OR and anesthesia teams, and oversees their performance. The OR and anesthesia teams have separate responsibilities, each responsibility involving around-the-clock support of planned and emergency equipment needs for a widely dispersed set of buildings.

To help improve outcomes of ES services, I established a set of objectives, as listed in Sidebar 7-1 (above).

Method

Before collecting data, I conducted an investigation to identify the PSFs. Once more, thinking in terms of a *systems* approach, I considered what *factors* could be affecting overall system performance. For example, could hints of interpersonal tensions be indicative of underlying systems problems? Could accepted practices or procedures be at odds with job descriptions, performance evaluation criteria, or policies? Does supervision have the means and opportunity to oversee performance? Do job descriptions and performance evaluations support or legitimize that activity? The PSFs identified at the onset are by no means final; more would be developed as work continued. In this case, I started with the considerations listed in Sidebar 7-2 (page 111).

To meet the study objectives, I interviewed OR "customers," primarily nurses and some physicians, as well as equipment staff and their managers, regarding task requirements, and identified system issues that affect success both within and beyond control of the ES technician team members. More specifically, I conducted the following seven tasks:

1. Determined requirements of the ES technicians to ensure availability and condition of equipment
2. Identified the functions assigned to personnel
3. Delineated the roles and duties of individuals per job descriptions and perceived operational expectations

> **Sidebar 7-2. Preliminary Considerations for Performance-Shaping Factors for the Equipment Supply Project**
>
> 1. The degree to which policies and procedures support performance
> 2. Changes in deployment of equipment (e.g., assignments of an airway emergency cart to a new area)
> 3. Communication issues
>   a. Technical issues such as effectiveness of the paging system
>   b. Communication of responsibilities across teams and for given areas and time periods
> 4. Perceptions of task prioritization
> 5. Skill set distribution between operating room (OR) and anesthesia equipment teams
> 6. Workload patterns (peaks and valleys) and distribution of work between anesthesia and surgery equipment specialist technicians
> 7. Conflicting perceptions of roles and responsibilities regarding delivery, setup and assistance with OR medical devices
> 8. Reactive versus proactive approach to equipment maintenance
> 9. Quantity of personnel and coverage during nights or when staff is on vacation
> 10. Effectiveness of supervision (e.g., oversight and auditing schedules)
>
> **Source:** The John Hopkins Hospital, Baltimore. Used with permission.

4. Analyzed and documented tasks and work processes with stakeholders
5. Identified constraints staff must work around
6. Reviewed paging records for timing performance of the paging system and response of those paged
7. Reviewed the computer-based tools used by the equipment manager for daily placement of equipment in the ORs

An important aspect of a human factors analysis of PSFs is that during the investigation phase, individuals may demonstrate defensiveness regarding their job performance. The human factors engineer may be met with doubt and even outright rejection by some stakeholders, inhibiting opportunities to identify improvements. However, by establishing rapport with each of the team members early on, treating all with respect, ensuring confidentiality, and resolving system problems that degrade one's ability to perform well, the human factors engineer will usually find that defensiveness tends to quickly disappear. In fact, as the stakeholders understand the purpose of the project, they tend to welcome the resulting removal of barriers to task completion and subsequently more congenial relationships are established between staff members.

Resulting Recommendations

The human factors analysis of PSFs led to a number of recommendations, which are now provided.

Changes to Job Descriptions and Performance Evaluation Criteria

Team member roles, responsibilities, and task priorities were more explicitly defined in the job descriptions to be more consistent with performance requirements. For example, the requirement to provide more proactive support of equipment was included, time expectations for completion of emergency tasks were documented qualitatively, and notice was provided that documentation supporting inventory and equipment checks would be audited. In addition, performance evaluation criteria were revised to identify emergency communication duties as a primary job function, and changes were made in performance assessment weightings for specific responsibilities.

Task Allocations

I recommended a review of the allocations of tasks between anesthesia and surgery ES technicians as well as among ES technicians, nurses, critical care technicians, and others. For example, I made the following recommendations:

1. Anesthesia ES technicians may be able to assume more administrative duties such as documentation, cart checks, and planning for in-service training.
2. Specific ES technicians could develop expertise on specific equipment to share duties across the expanding number of medical devices requiring specific skills.
3. Nurses rather than ES technicians could operate lasers in ORs because the only task is to switch the laser between standby and on.
4. ES technicians in one of the buildings could process their own carts on weekends.
5. Clinical engineering now assumes the role of performing and documenting daily anesthesia preoperative machine checks to avoid role confusion.

Team Coordination

It was recommended that decisions regarding emergency-airway cart contents, placement, labeling, and access be made in a forum that included the stakeholders designated by a multidisciplinary perioperative services team. Furthermore, because the equipment manager and ES technicians are responsible for cart condition and contents, nursing's safety audits of carts should be conducted in the presence of an equipment representative. I also recommended that critical care technicians and other OR staff be aware of the need to inform ES technicians what equipment has been displaced and what repairs may be needed. ES staff should feel empowered to report discrepancies in this important information trail. All these actions should enable better tracking and availability of equipment.

Communication

To ensure that ES technicians respond to requests for resupply of emergency carts that were made by pager, the pager number was added to an equipment manager's pager. Managers verify that the request was met and that the loop was closed. To further verify that electronic communications are reliable and acted on, the equipment manager's supervisor and I recommended that the equipment manager conduct paging drills and document both paging system performance and timing of responses.

Training

To address training, which is generally viewed as the most important means to ensure the technical competency of staff, the equipment manager rescheduled training activities to enable delivery of more intense training to smaller groups and to allow better checks of technical competency. To promote understanding of the challenges that ES technicians face in meeting equipment needs, it was recommended that clinicians also be educated about those challenges.

CHAPTER 7
Human Factors Engineering at The Johns Hopkins Hospital

Supervision

Equipment availability can be affected by some surgeons' practice of double-booking devices so they can later decide which to use—a practice that can lead to shortages for other ORs. To better plan equipment scheduling across ORs, an equipment summary form was developed to identify total numbers of specific equipment needed across and not just within ORs. The equipment manager can now run checks for double-booking before disseminating requirements for the next-day equipment.

Other Improvements

In addition to the recommendations and actions described, the equipment manager initiated the following improvements:

1. Adaptation of two computers on wheels for inspecting and documenting inventory on airway carts, video carts, and other equipment
2. Expansion of staffing classifications to include a career ladder with three rather than two perioperative ES technician levels to better identify roles and provide more opportunity for advancement
3. Development of improved ES technician competency tests and equipment checklists
4. Daily assignment of scope-cleaning responsibilities to one person for better control of those activities
5. Development of a means to verify performance of hourly OR equipment checks while OR procedures are in process

Summary

The results of this study included, among other improvements, establishment of more cohesive teams whose members had better definition of their roles and responsibilities, a better means to evaluate technicians against explicitly defined performance criteria, and better use of tools for communicating equipment needs and documenting equipment condition.

REFLECTIONS

When performing safety analyses, consider that whatever their differences, FTA and FMEA are used to identify conditions that lead to hazards and opportunities for improvements. In each case, the exercise involves systems thinking to identify the many conditions or factors that can affect system performance. This is why learning about HFE can greatly bolster systems thinking and increase one's proficiency as a patient safety advocate.

One clear benefit that the human factors engineer brings to the health care organization is the freedom from clinical responsibilities. This enables him or her to focus solely on comprehensive analyses, in which a series of "What if?" questions are posed to address all possible systems issues. Such questions might include: "Was there anything in the count bucket from the last case before the first sponge was thrown in?" or "Why is it necessary to post handwritten instructions near equipment to promote proper use?" Yet, as discussed in other chapters (Chapters 6 and 8), the human factors engineer can teach HFE thinking and skills sets to clinicians and administrators so that they, too, can apply HFE tools to improve patient safety. Administrators and clinicians who are interested in how human factors can affect patient safety are probably already curious and analytic by nature and thus well-suited to employ some of the steps listed in Sidebar 7-3 (page 114) to promote patient safety.

One challenge that your organization may confront while improving patient safety is that the number of opportunities for improvement almost always exceeds the resources available to address them. Therefore, you may find it difficult to choose which projects to pursue. In making such decisions, it may help to determine the feasibility of implementing candidate solutions that have a beneficial impact on safe-

> **Sidebar 7-3. Human Factors Engineering (HFE)–Type Steps that Clinicians and Administrators Can Take to Promote Patient Safety**
>
> 1. Identify unsafe conditions by evaluating near misses and watching proactively for opportunities for harm.
> 2. Analyze the contributing factors using systems thinking as taught in HFE in health care courses.
> 3. Test the observations in safe conditions to see if the contributing factors may indeed cause an undesired effect.
> 4. Log unsafe conditions as hazards or failure modes according to severity level and probability using the risk-assessment criteria shown in Table 7-4 (page 115).
> 5. Determine feasibility and practicality of resolving each issue.
> 6. Prioritize your efforts accordingly.
> 7. Track the hazards in the log, noting status through the resolution process as open, monitor (solution agreed on but not implemented), or closed (implemented).
> 8. Insist that an organizational process be used to reconcile conflicts that affect safety by relying on the evaluation and judgment of management to provide guidance where differences cannot be resolved.
>
> **Source:** The John Hopkins Hospital, Baltimore. Used with permission.

ty. Feasibility analyses conducted early in the analysis phase of studies can help identify not only which solutions should be pursued but which projects have the best potential for reducing harm. (For more discussion of feasibility analysis and other systems-analysis techniques, see Blanchard.[5]) By contrast, we did not conduct feasibility analyses in either Case Study 1 or 2 because the issues were considered sufficiently important to benefit from any means of improvement.

In my three years' experience in applying HFE methods in the health care industry, I have learned that there is ample opportunity for improvement in device design, training, procedures, and processes. For example, at JHH we have identified 76 devices with alarms that can be used at the bedside and more than 300 devices used in the OR. Although we cannot change device design in the short term, opportunities exist to work hand in hand with clinicians and vendors to influence future improvements. One of the more striking things I have learned is the high degree of motivation and interest clinicians have in participating in safety improvements by identifying safety issues and working closely with diverse teams to resolve them. A human factors engineer or other HFE professional adds another perspective to these challenges by helping to identify unique obstacles to safety and criteria for their remediation. For those who do not have ready access to HFE expertise, there are excellent references for learning HFE methods and standards (*see* the Appendix to Part I, pages 71–75).

Table 7-4. Assessing Acceptability of Risk by Probability and Severity*

Probability Level	Severity Level				
	Negligible	Minor	Serious	Critical	Catastrophic
Frequent	▓	▓	▓	▓	▓
Probable	▓	▓	▓	▓	▓
Occasional			▓	▓	▓
Remote				▓	▓
Improbable					

Key:

▓ Unacceptable risk

☐ Acceptable risk

* Cited in Sidebar 7-3 (page 114).

Source: American National Standards Institute/Association for the Advancement of Medical Instrumentation/International Standardization Organization (ANSI/AAMI/ISO) 14971: *Application of Risk Management to Medical Devices.* Arlington, VA: AAMI, 2007. Used with permission.

A final thought. Providing direct patient care offers more immediate gratification than patient safety projects do. In the former, concrete results of your actions are seen relatively quickly. In the latter, good results require data collection over extended periods, perhaps followed by refinement, more performance measurement, and challenges associated with effecting organizational or design change. Perseverance in these efforts is key to realizing the gratification. Remember that while the results of patient safety efforts may not necessarily be immediately seen with individual patients, they do provide benefits that impact a large population.

References

1. University of Maryland, Department of Computer Science, The Museum of User Interfaces: *Alphonse Chapanis, 1917–2002.* http://www.cs.umd.edu/hcil/muiseum/chapanis/chapanis_page.htm (accessed Apr. 12, 2010).
2. Approved American National Standard ANSI Z535.4-2007: *American National Standard for Product Safety Signs and Labels,* (Jun. 1, 2007). http://www.nema.org/stds/complimentary-docs/upload/ANSI_Z535.4-2007_WEB-2.pdf (accessed Apr. 12, 2010).
3. ECRI Institute: *News Release: ECRI Institute Issues "Top Ten Health Technology Hazards for 2010,"* Dec. 2, 2009. https://www.ecri.org/Press/Pages/2010_Top_Ten_Health_Technology_Hazards.aspx (accessed Apr. 12, 2010).
4. U.S. Nuclear Regulatory Commission: *Fault Tree Handbook* (NUREG 0492), Jan. 1981. Office of Nuclear Regulatory Research. http://www.nrc.gov/reading-rm/doc-collections/nuregs/staff/sr0492/ (accessed Apr. 12, 2010).
5. Blanchard B.S.: *Systems Engineering Management,* 3rd ed. Hoboken, NJ: John Wiley and Sons, 2004.

CHAPTER 8

Applying Human Factors Engineering in a Patient Safety and Quality Program

Laurie D. Wolf, M.S., C.P.E., A.S.Q.-C.S.S.B.B.

MY HUMAN FACTORS ENGINEERING JOURNEY TO HEALTH CARE

With a master's degree in human factors engineering (HFE) in hand, I found my first job, in advanced vehicle engineering, at General Motors (Pontiac, Michigan), which exposed me to an industrial environment and provided experience in product design, usability assessment, and auditory displays. After three years I went to work in the electronics and space division for Emerson Electric (St. Louis), where, working on various military contracts, I had the opportunity to design control panels and hand controllers and to perform detailed task analyses as needed to support design decisions and improve processes. My projects always involved military personnel who were young, physically fit, and highly motivated and had relatively similar anthropometric values (body dimensions), strengths, and abilities. After five years, I began searching for opportunities to work with a more diverse population. I saw in health care the opportunity to address extreme diversity and culture barriers in both patients and caregivers.

After I became interested in the health care environment—with its varied human factors possibilities—I developed a subspecialty in injury prevention.

In 1993 BJC Corporate Health Services, a division of BJC HealthCare that was interested in creating a new revenue stream by providing injury-prevention consulting, hired me to help local companies accommodate returning injured employees. I trained therapists to consider not just biomechanics but also a wide range of issues, such as noise, lighting, and wasted motions. Later, we branched out into more proactive projects in improving productivity and efficiency and decreasing the risk of musculoskeletal injury.

In my 16 years at BJC HealthCare, my numerous projects have involved a wide variety of human factors, such as usability (for example, safety needles, intravenous pumps), mental workload capability, interruptions, equipment (for example, control and display) design, workstation layout, glare/lighting, and noise assessments. To prepare for process improvement work with caregivers, I achieved Black Belt certification in Six Sigma and have spent the last four years using HFE methodology to focus on patient safety.

FROM INJURY PREVENTION TO PROCESS IMPROVEMENT AT THE BJC HEALTHCARE SYSTEM

BJC HealthCare is a large, nonprofit health care organization, employing 26,622 people in 13 health care institutions throughout Missouri and Illinois. It provides services to urban, suburban, and rural communities in inpatient and outpatient care, primary care, community health and wellness, workplace health, home health, community mental health, rehabilitation, long term care, and hospice. BJC HealthCare, the largest nongovernmental employer in Missouri, is affiliated with Washington University School of Medicine. Barnes-Jewish Hospital is a 1,200-bed academic medical center located in St. Louis, with a Lean transformation team that is working to change culture, standardize work flows, and improve processes for more than 9,000 employees, 800 residents and 1,700 physicians, 1,106 staffed beds, and 55,000 admissions annually.

Beginning with Injury Prevention

In my work as an injury-prevention consultant, I spent three years in collecting and presenting industry stories that successfully decreased workers' compensation costs and increased productivity. During this time, BJC experienced an increase in workers' compensation costs and asked us to develop a program that would decrease injuries and save worker's compensation costs for the entire organization. In 1996 an interdisciplinary team—from human resources, safety, nursing, housekeeping, food services, occupational health, risk management, and other entities throughout BJC HealthCare—met to discuss and design a program to promote employee health. Data for work-related injuries indicated that musculoskeletal led all other work-related injuries in time lost from work (a measurement of severity) and that body-substance exposures (primarily from needlesticks) had the greatest potential for life-changing or even life-ending outcomes for employees. To promote employee health, we developed a three-pronged approach (*see* Sidebar 8-1, page 119) and created a program—BJC WellAware—to plan, execute, and coordinate efforts. Interventions were designed to lower workers' compensation expenses, with the savings used to fund general wellness initiatives.

By creating one evidence-based source of expertise for ergonomic initiatives we accomplished the following:

- Presented ergonomics as a science to a community that respects scientific research and application
- Standardized policy and practice
- Minimized concurrent nonstandard efforts
- Established the program as a national model

In one initiative, for example, we established a vetting process for products designed to minimize effort of nurses in handling patients. Implementing patient-lift devices in long term care facilities to enable employees to safely transfer patients in and out of bed reduced patient lifting–related injuries by 60% and workers' compensation costs by 45% in less than three years, with continuing success. As our reputation for scientific evaluation of products grew, standardization throughout the system became easier. This standardization reduced wasted resources at each facility and resulted in the implementation of more effective and often more economical solutions. We also undertook more subtle interventions without considerable monetary investment to eliminate sources of slips, trips, falls, or strains for BJC employees.

For example, we established a hotline to report potentially dangerous walk areas or other sites of impending injury and posted signs to educate and promote employee awareness, owner-

> ## Sidebar 8-1. A Three-Pronged Approach to Improve Employee Health
>
> **Ergonomics**
> - Established one human factors engineering–skilled authority for ergonomic expertise to promote practical application of evidence-based, systematic, and scientific methodology*
> - Created a team of specialists (with education equivalent of physical therapy assistants) trained to perform standard assessments, interventions, education, and process improvements*
>
> **Infection Prevention**
> - Analyzed the frequency and severity of employee body-substance exposures
> - Created a 24-hours-a-day, 7-days-a-week, body-substance-exposure hotline for assessment, referral, and timely treatment with prophylactic medication
>
> **Wellness**
> - Established a health-risk assessment to provide individuals with information and to provide the system with aggregate data of basic wellness information
> - Provided health fairs for employees to know their numbers related to blood pressure, body mass index, cholesterol, and blood sugar levels
>
> *For the first nine years, I fulfilled this role.
>
> **Source:** BJC HealthCare, St. Louis. Used with permission.

ship, and participation. Another awareness factor involved a study of employee shoe choice to suggest recommendations on what type of shoe provided the best traction for workers on a typical hospital-flooring material. In an easy-to-implement intervention, plastic umbrella sleeves were made available at hospital doorways to keep drips from forming slippery surfaces for both visitors and employees.

In 2008 our injury-prevention program received recognition in Canada, serving as a model for a pilot program in six hospitals. The Ontario Safety Association for Community and Healthcare received funding from the Ontario Neurotrauma Foundation to set up an ergonomic framework to prevent slips, trips, falls, and musculoskeletal disorders in health care.

The Need for HFE Expertise in Process Improvement

Many successful process improvements in quality and patient safety were achieved with traditional continuous improvement methodologies, such as the Plan-Do-Check-Act cycle. However, some of the projects may not have reached the desired goals or had difficulty sustaining improvements because of a lack of consideration of the human factors and a systems approach to improvement. According to the Systems Engineering Initiative for Patient Safety (SEIPS) model, a systems approach entails five interdependent aspects: (1) all tasks to be performed, (2) the caregivers performing the tasks, (3) the technology or tools used, (4) the environment, and (5) the organization.[1]

This systems approach enabled us to study

issues such as incorrect programming of an intravenous (IV) pump, which involved the use of a calculator to determine appropriate dosages; low light levels in a patient's room during medicine administration; interruptions that constantly occur in the medicine-preparation area; and even the mental workload of a nurse before, during, and after an error. This experience broadened the BJC perspective on how errors occur and how HFE methods could improve patient safety.

Using Lean Six Sigma

In 2004 BJC began using Lean Six Sigma techniques to supplement its performance improvement structure under its Center for Healthcare Quality and Effectiveness (now called the Center for Clinical Excellence). In 2005 it began a formal rollout of an enterprisewide Lean Six Sigma effort. Barnes-Jewish Hospital has worked to combine the power of Lean Six Sigma principles and tools to reduce defects and process variability and enhance the efficiency and quality of key care delivery and support processes. Lean Six Sigma techniques, which embody the principles of industrial engineering, complement HFE methodology.

My Six Sigma black belt project addressed the discharge process for mothers and their newborn on the women and infants division at the hospital. The project's goal was to get patients discharged earlier in the day so that beds would be available for new patients, preventing backup in the emergency department and in labor and delivery. By changing the discharge process and the way physicians conducted discharge rounding and procedures, we were able to improve the percentage of mothers and babies who were discharged by 11:00 P.M. (13:00) from 0% to 87%. The discharge project was one of several projects involved in a value stream analysis that resulted in the reduction of adverse safety events from nine to one in almost two years, also resulting in a cost avoidance of $1.3 million.

APPLYING HFE IN A PATIENT SAFETY AND QUALITY PROGRAM

In 2006 the vice president for patient safety and quality recognized the need for a human factors expert among her team of management engineers. When I transferred to Barnes-Jewish Hospital's patient safety and quality department, the team included members with backgrounds in nursing, business, and mechanical engineering. The hospital was committed to using a systems approach to analyzing problems and agreed that including HFE methodology to develop solutions was critical to success. Leadership understood the necessity of considering humans' interaction with their tools and environment when trying to mistake-proof patient care practices. During my first year at the hospital, I developed a four-hour human factors module with the BJC team, which is presented as Case Study 1.

Case Study 1. A Human Factors Module

The goal of developing the module was to increase awareness of human factors methodology and provide tools that could be applied to problem solving. This module was incorporated into the nonconsecutive, four-week Six Sigma black belt training program that continues to be offered in-house to BJC employees and medical staff. Participants attend one week of class and then return to their normal work activities for three weeks with "homework" to achieve milestones on a Six Sigma project of their choice before returning to the next week of classroom training. The human factors module is typically scheduled during the third week of training.

The human factors module, which is provided two or three times per year, combines a lecture format with hands-on workshop activities in which the attendees have the opportunity to apply HFE checklists to their Six Sigma projects. Each year, I update the lecture with projects I have worked on in the previous year that demonstrate interesting human factors principles. The module begins with an introduction to HFE principles and discussion about the role that human factors has in health care. Considering human factors helps us to understand how a person interacts with the equipment needed to perform a job task. Several examples of problems and the human factors solution are shown in photographs and illustrated by stories of actual events that have occurred in health care. Time is allotted for the class to discuss human factors issues in their own black belt projects and brainstorm solutions. This exercise also allows the class to practice completing the human factors checklists to enable them to understand areas of concern that may require intervention. The objective of this module is for attendees to bring human factors knowledge back to their work area so that they can use it to address problems. Selected topics covered in the module are listed in Sidebar 8-2 (page 122).

Case studies are now presented to describe sample improvement projects, ranging from equipment design to culture change, that have involved HFE issues and required multidisciplinary collaboration to ensure success. Whereas some projects were short, requiring only a few hours to complete (Case Study 4), others were very complex and required months to design and implement (Case Studies 2 and 3).

Case Study 2. Improving Medical Equipment Availability by Decentralizing Cleaning

In 2007 the vice president for patient safety and quality asked me to help facilitate a Lean Six Sigma project, which involved wasted motions, to address nurses' frustration in obtaining IV pumps. The solution would require a dramatic change in process. The primary goal was to enhance patient safety by reducing equipment delivery time and the time nurses spent in attempting to locate equipment. The initial scope of the project was to improve the availability of IV pumps, but the scope was expanded to apply to other equipment after the process proved to be a success. Sponsorship for the project came from top administration, with further support found throughout various disciplines and departments. The patient care director served as the project's executive sponsor, and a clinical nurse specialist conducted the project as part of her Six Sigma class work. The project team also included nurses; clinical nurse managers; unit secretaries and representatives from information services, receiving, central sterile processing, and materials supply. An essential partner in this project was our IV pump supplier.

Before the Intervention

Before the intervention, the broken process resulted in a classic work-around by nursing staff. In the case of IV pumps, nurses would be fast to claim a pump from a discharged patient's room, do an unplanned quick cleaning that may vary from the precise steps and sterilization dry-time process that are conducted by the trained equipment suppliers—and use the pump for their just-admitted patient. Or they would go to a neighboring unit to "borrow" a pump without really intending to return it. Needless to say, nurses were extremely frustrated regarding the lack of readily available equipment.

The equipment supply partners and their employees also had frustrations. The employees were required to retrieve, clean, and deliver patient equipment, moving it back and forth from the centralized cleaning area in the basement, as much as a half mile, up to the nursing divisions. There were long elevator waits going up and coming back down. They had to awk-

> ## Sidebar 8-2. Selected Topics Covered in the Human Factors Module
>
> - Introduction: Define human factors engineering (HFE) and how it applies to health care and the multidisciplinary approach
> - Consequences of human error
> - Human capabilities and limitations: Fitting work to the worker
> - Human reliability
> - HFE and purchasing decisions: Return on investment
> - Benefits of HFE in health care
> - Systems approach (3 components: organization, human, environment; *see* Figure 8-1, page 123).
> - Organizational component of the system approach
>   - Administrative issues: sharp/blunt end of accident investigation
>   - Medication error story that illustrates the Swiss cheese model*
>   - Training
> - Human component of the system approach
>   - Physical aspects: Anthropometry and physical design
>   - Endurance, force, and fatigue
>   - Human cognitive capabilities: working memory
>   - Mental workload
>   - Human perceptual capabilities: Auditory examples
>   - Desensitization phenomenon (e.g., alarm fatigue)
>   - Visual perception: Illumination, visibility
>   - Look-alike, sound-alike risks
> - Environmental component of the systems approach
>   - Design layout: work area, medicine preparation area, patient room, supply rooms
>   - Equipment design
>   - Supply design solutions: medication packaging, location separation issues
> - Summary and action-item assignment
>
> * Reason J.: *Managing the Risks of Organizational Accidents*. Burlington, VT: Ashgate Publishing Company, 2000.
>
> **Source:** BJC HealthCare, St. Louis. Used with permission.

wardly maneuver lots of equipment at one time, resulting in the use of poor body mechanics. In addition, everyone had concerns about transporting used patient equipment through public areas, risking potential exposure to visitors and staff. Soiled-equipment rooms were unorganized, making it difficult to know what equipment needed to be cleaned (*see* Figure 8-2, page 124).

A One-Day Event

The first phase of this project was conducted as a one-day event. The clinical nurse specialist and I took about two weeks for preparation. The event had to be planned one month in advance to ensure that the multidisciplinary participants were able to attend. During the event, the team developed an intervention that was pilot tested in one patient care area for two weeks.

CHAPTER 8
Applying Human Factors Engineering in a Patient Safety and Quality Program

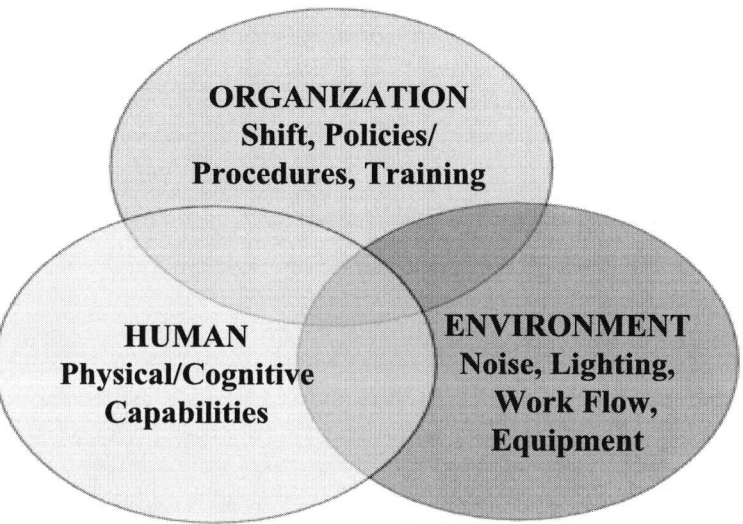

Figure 8-1. Components of a Human Factors Engineering Systems Approach

The overlap areas in this Venn diagram among the three components—organization, human, and environment—indicate the need to for a comprehensive approach to identifying and addressing human factors engineering issues.

Source: BJC HealthCare, St. Louis. Used with permission.

During the one-day event, a combination of Lean Six Sigma and HFE tools were used. A task analysis was performed to understand the current process for getting equipment to a patient, cleaning it after use, and getting it ready for the next patient. The current state was illustrated in a process map so that all participants could understand the required tasks and roles of everyone involved. The process began with the nurse ordering an IV pump, then the next steps were listed, such as equipment supplier receiving order and delivering pump to requesting nurse, nurse using pump to deliver medication, nurse discontinuing use and returning it to the soiled-equipment room and then transporting to decontamination. The process ended with cleaning the pump and preparing for next use. The group then took a "field trip" to walk the entire process to see where each activity was performed. Each process step was reviewed to see if it was value added or non–value added. Time estimates were determined for each process step.

Next, a fishbone diagram (*see* Figure 8-3, page 125) was developed to understand the reasons why equipment (such as an IV pump) was not available in a timely manner. For example, equipment could not be found in the computerized order entry system; equipment was not properly prepared by nurses, so equipment supplier personnel were not allowed to take the equipment for cleaning; and nurses were not told when the equipment arrived and therefore

Figure 8-2. The Soiled-Equipment Room Before and After the Intervention

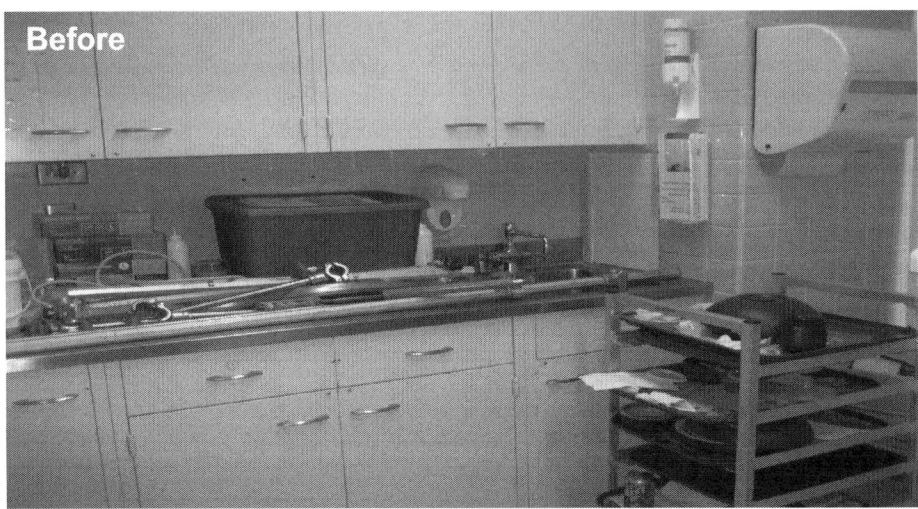

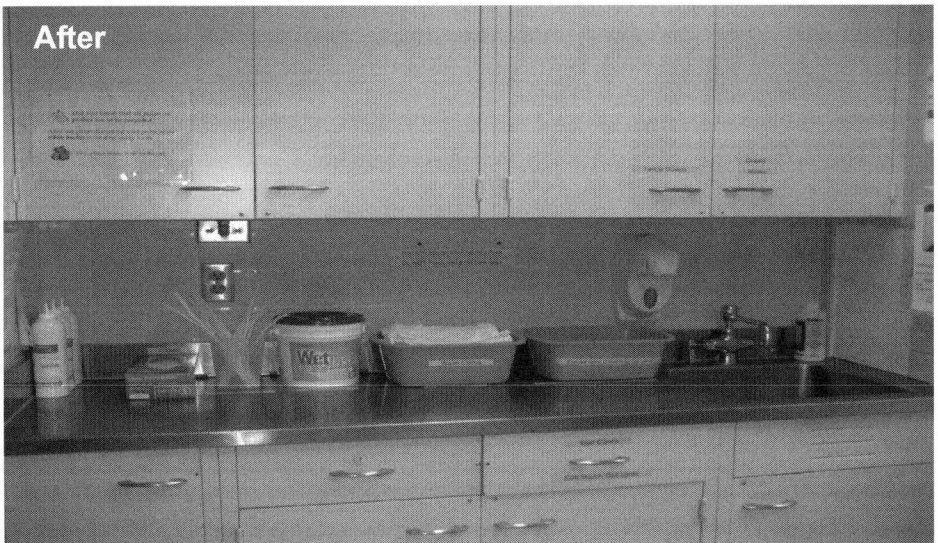

Before the intervention, the soiled-equipment room was unorganized, and there was no room for cleaning supplies (top photo). After the intervention, the soiled-equipment room was clearly marked with space for equipment that needed cleaning, and appropriate supplies were readily available (bottom photo). A color version of this figure is also provided online (http:/www.jcrinc.com/UHFE10/extras).

Source: BJC HealthCare, St. Louis. Used with permission.

CHAPTER 8
Applying Human Factors Engineering in a Patient Safety and Quality Program

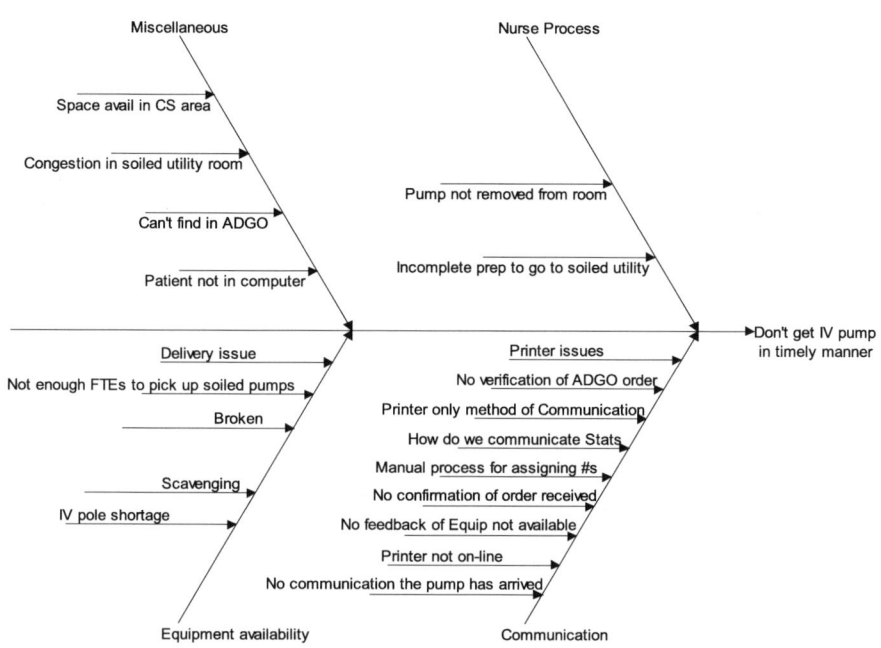

Figure 8-3. Fishbone Diagram on Reasons Why Equipment Not Available in a Timely Manner

This fishbone diagram was developed to determine the reasons why equipment (such as an intravenous pump) was not available in a timely manner. CS, Central Sterile; ADGO, computerized equipment ordering system; FTE, full-time equivalent; IV, intravenous.

Source: BJC HealthCare, St. Louis. Used with permission.

were not aware that it was available. As shown in Figure 8-4 (page 126), the numerous reasons were grouped into the following categories: communication, equipment availability, and nursing process (for example, nurse forgot to remove tubing from the pump).

The future state required the equipment to be cleaned on the nursing division in the soiled-equipment room and then placed in the clean-equipment storage area ready for next use, as shown in Figure 8-5 (page 127). This challenged the team to determine how many IV pumps must be stored on each division to ensure that a pump is available at all times.

Intervention

This critical element of the new process involved setting up and maintaining "par levels" of equipment on specific divisions based on usage. To do this, the team approached unit leadership with an empowering request: How many clean IV pumps would you need on-hand to avoid ever calling downstairs for pump deliv-

125

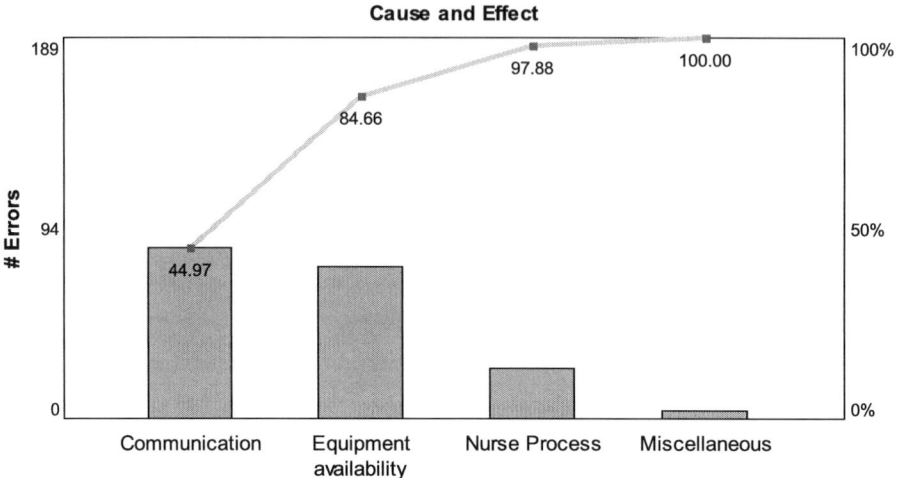

Figure 8-4. Pareto Diagram Showing Four Categories of Reasons Why Equipment Not Available

The four categories of reasons why equipment was not available in a timely manner, as determined by the fishbone diagram (Figure 8-3, page 125), cumulatively accounted for 100% of the cases.

Source: BJC HealthCare, St. Louis. Used with permission.

ery? Initially, the par levels were set to this requested amount, and then adjusted as usage patterns were observed. One challenge was to balance the number of available IV pumps with the timing of the cleaning process. A two-hour rounding schedule was set up by the equipment supplier; an employee visited each division at least every two hours to check if there was any equipment that needed to be cleaned. Typically, he or she would find that the original par level estimate was too high and that the number could be reduced after it was apparent that the nurses trusted that they would always have a pump available when it was needed.

The "5S" (sort, set in order, shine, standardize, sustain) technique[2] was used in every soiled- and clean-equipment room to prepare an appropriate space for the new cleaning process. This technique organizes an area so it is easy to use by all employees and makes any problems obvious. Visual cues, such as red tape on the floor, indicate the proper space for the dirty equipment. A designated cleaning area (approximately 3 ft. × 2 ft.) was labeled and stocked with the appropriate supplies. The tape on the floor in both the clean- and soiled-equipment rooms designates the proper location, as determined by the lead charge nurse, and the amount of clean equipment available. The configuration varied according to the building layout of each division. The cleaning supplies were maintained by the unit secretary and housekeeping staff. The visual cues made it obvious when there was too much equipment in need of cleaning or not enough clean equipment available to fill the par levels.

CHAPTER 8
Applying Human Factors Engineering in a Patient Safety and Quality Program

Figure 8-5. Decentralized Equipment Cleaning Cycle

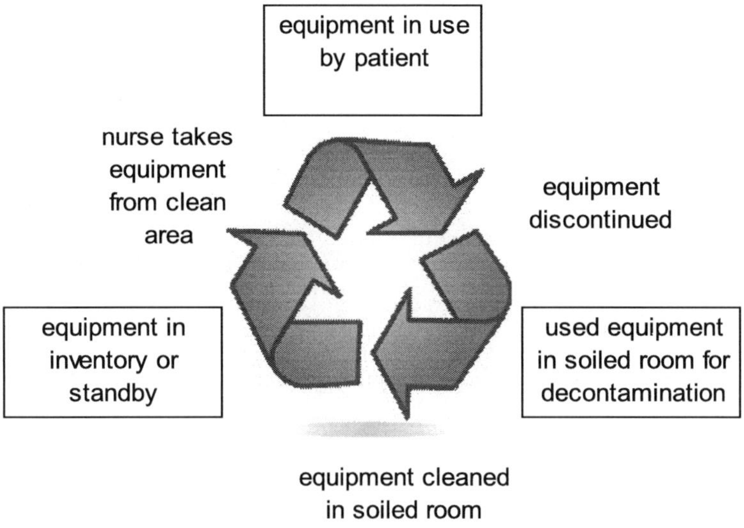

- equipment in use by patient
- equipment discontinued
- used equipment in soiled room for decontamination
- equipment cleaned in soiled room
- equipment in inventory or standby
- nurse takes equipment from clean area

The future state required the equipment to be cleaned on the nursing division in the soiled-equipment room and then placed in the clean-equipment storage area ready for next use, as shown.

Source: BJC HealthCare, St. Louis. Used with permission.

The preintervention photo (Figure 8-6a, page 128) shows a shower chair, IV pole, cart, and trash can in no particular order. As shown in the postintervention photo (Figure 8-6b, page 128), areas were indicated with red tape and labels to indicate where each type of equipment belonged.

Spread

After the patient care staff indicated that they wanted to make the two-week intervention permanent, the patient care operations supervisor rolled out the intervention across the entire hospital, one division at a time, until acceptance was achieved. She also partnered with the regional manager of the equipment supplier to address issues identified during the rollout and for sustaining the new process.

Results

Since the intervention was rolled out throughout the entire Barnes-Jewish Hospital, the wait time for equipment has improved considerably. The time to obtain an IV pump ranged from 40 minutes to 4 hours 36 minutes (mean, 2 hours 7 minutes). With the new par levels, the wait time is completely eliminated. In addition, the rate of lost equipment decreased almost in half, from 12% to 6.9%.

Reflections

The concept of decentralizing equipment cleaning required employees to build trust. The new process was implemented on one volunteer division as a two-week trial. It was so successful that the division did not want the trial to end, and several divisions, hearing about the positive results, wanted to be selected next. The new

Figure 8-6. Soiled-Equipment Room, Pre- and Postintervention

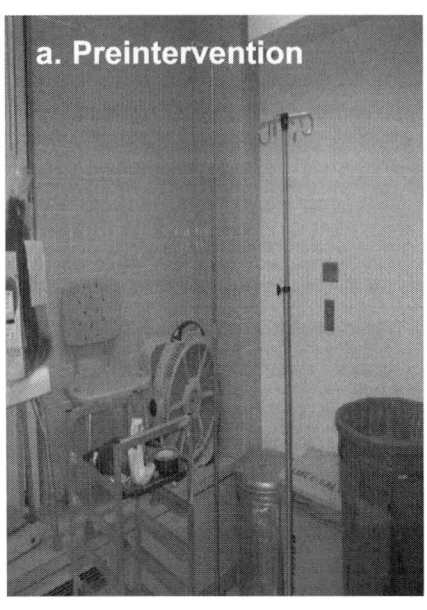
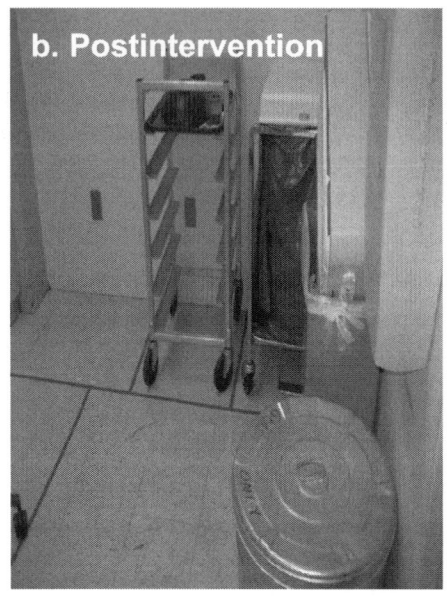

Lack of organization made it difficult to find equipment (left). Used equipment is placed appropriately, ready to be cleaned (right). A color version of this figure is also provided online (http://www.jcrinc.com/UHFE10/extras).

Source: BJC HealthCare, St. Louis. Used with permission.

process has now been in place for the entire 1,200-bed hospital for more than two years. The equipment supplier has expanded the program to include other equipment, such as bedside commodes, sequential compressive devices, walkers, bed checks, portable suction, and bariatric equipment.

This project empowered multiple disciplines to work together and partner with an outside supplier to create the best possible system for all. The results demonstrate how even a "low-tech" solution with minimal capital expense can generate sustainable improvements in service delivery and tremendous gains in staff satisfaction. As one nurse described it, the project was a true gift to nurses, the "best process improvement" she had seen in 30 years.

Case Study 3. Inpatient Medicine Process Improvements

Originally, we tried to recruit a physician with Lean Six Sigma and HFE skills to lead a process improvement initiative on 13 inpatient medicine divisions. After an unsuccessful nationwide search in 2007, I was selected by the chief medical officer to facilitate the physicians in this effort, and I partnered with a physician, the patient safety fellow, to help me understand the medical processes as needed.

Excellent physician engagement in the numerous process improvement projects has been achieved through flexibility about structuring meetings and improvement events around physician needs and availability. Tools are applied with ingenuity and flexibility to achieve their intended purpose but to succeed without disrupting patient care in a highly complex environment.

The methods and strategies we use for our improvements are guided by a steering committee, a multidisciplinary team lead by the chief medical officer and that consists of medical physicians, an emergency room physician, chief medicine residents, vice president of patient care service/chief nurse executive, director of patient care, patient placement manager, director of medicine service, nurse managers, and an HFE engineer [L.D.W.]

This initiative, ongoing since 2007, has required 25%–75% of my time, depending on the type of activity. Typically, careful preparation for a process improvement event, which is critical to ensure the best usage of each physician's time, takes twice as long as the actual event. Generally, improvement tools are most successful if they are prepared and populated as much as possible before the event (with input from individual physicians). Such tools include the following:

- A Failure Mode and Effects Analysis, which is used to identify product or process problems before they occur[3]
- A link analysis, which is used to reveal the sequence of connections between two elements of an interface required to complete a task (either information or movement of a person or his or her limbs)[4]
- An impact matrix, which is used to evaluate a solution on the basis of the effort (ease of implementation) and impact (anticipated changes).[5] Such an evaluation helps to narrow the number of possible solutions to the most feasible for implementation.
- A cause-and-effect matrix, which is used to capture the Voice of the Customer and relate it to process input variables[2]

It is more time efficient to have physicians review and verify a process than develop it initially. Key stakeholders and sponsors are identified for each project to help prepare a first draft for steering committee review.

Value stream analysis was used to develop a plan for implementing several improvement projects. This analysis provides an understanding of the process steps required to admit, diagnose, treat, and discharge a patient. Areas for improvement were identified and provided a road map for future projects. Some of the improvement projects that were identified are now briefly described.

Emergency Department Communication to Admitting Physicians

Reason for Action: Improve handoff processes between emergency department (ED) and admitting services.

Solution: A medicine reconciliation process was "hardwired" into the ED admission procedure by adding questions into the documentation system. A summary report from the ED physician was organized according to the admitting physicians' needs to make information easier to find and to decrease the time needed to complete a history and physical on a newly admitted patient. A new admission process was also implemented that shifted the work of a medicine resident from triaging patients in the ED to admitting patients at night. A combination of all these projects reduced the length of stay in the ED by one hour when we compared the preintervention (January through April 2008) and postintervention (May through June 2008) periods, a statistically significant improvement

($p < .001$). This average of one-hour improvement continues to be sustained to this day.

Forms Required to Be Completed by a Physician

Reason for Action: Admission forms and process are different on each floor and difficult to find, and pages can be confused, causing incorrect patient identification.

Solution: An admission packet was developed with required forms preprinted with patient identification to increase patient safety by reducing the opportunity for patient identification errors. All forms needed by a physician are located in one place in the same arrangements on all 13 medicine floors. The time required to complete admit forms decreased by more than 50% during a simulation in which several physicians were randomly assigned two simulated cases and asked to complete paperwork to "admit" the two simulated patients using the traditional method. The experiment was completed again using the new process with two more simulated patients.

Transparent Plan of Care

Reason for Action: It is difficult to identify the physician, nurse, and plan of care for the patient.

Solution: A patient information board was placed inside the patient's room to show the physician, nurse, and plan of care for the patient each day. The census board in the nursing station was reorganized to show everyone which physician and nurse are responsible for each patient and their contact information. Discharge sheets that are completed by all residents at the end of each shift were made available electronically. This enabled all caregivers to review the plan of care for the patients for the upcoming shift.

Discharge Process

Reason for Action: Some 50% of the patients were discharged after 4 P.M. (16:00), causing a delay in admission of new patients

Solution: One solution was to encourage physician communication about "Anticipate Discharge Tomorrow." Communication for "Discharge home today" with the goal to discharge by 1:00 P.M. (13:00) was done by all patient care staff. A discharge planning board with a visual reminder of tasks to be completed before discharge is located in the staff area and updated daily.

A time line with the topics addressed in this value stream is shown in Figure 8-7 (page 131). Results of many of these projects have been communicated through articles in the physician newsletters, *Spotlight on Patient Safety and Quality*, e-mails, and presentations at physician meetings and executive out-briefs. Results have been shared with other hospitals through papers, presentations, and posters at national conferences.

By the time I found out about the following case, the clinical engineering department had already found a solution and were in the process of implementing the changes. Consequently, it took no preparation or time on my part.

Case Study 4. Nitrogen Oxide (N_2O) Connected to Carbon Dioxide (CO_2) Outlet

In 2009 the hospital's chief medical officer made me aware of an event in the operating room (OR) that involved incorrect tube connections. The hardest part of this project for me was finding out who was working on it. After several calls I found the correct department—clinical engineering—that had already addressed the problem. All I did was go to the area and take photographs before and after the intervention.

According to clinical engineering, the physician who asked the technician to connect the N_2O, was unaware that the headwall in this particular

CHAPTER 8
Applying Human Factors Engineering in a Patient Safety and Quality Program

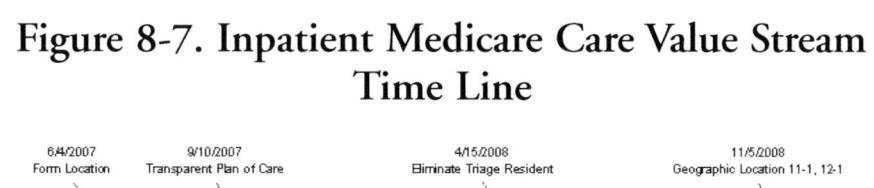
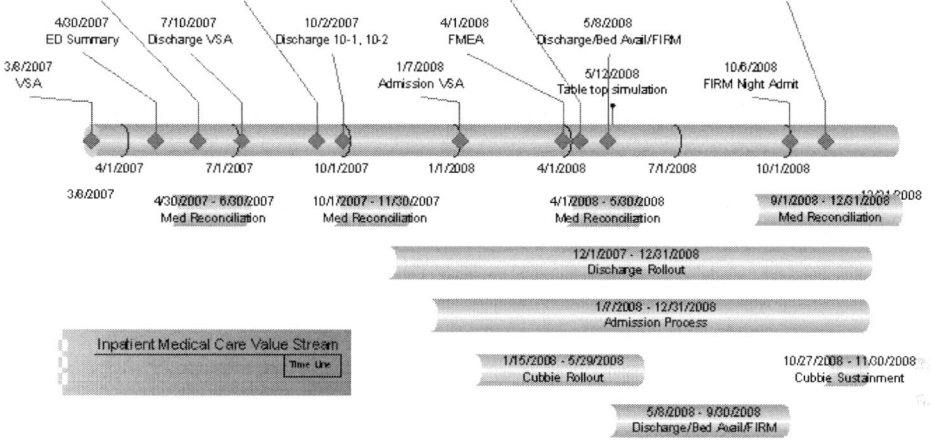

Figure 8-7. Inpatient Medicare Care Value Stream Time Line

The time line shows the topics and durations of the process improvement projects. VSA, value stream analysis. A color version of this figure is also provided online (http://www.jcrinc.com/UHFE10/extras).

Source: BJC HealthCare, St. Louis. Used with permission.

OR, unlike most of the other ORs, headwall did not have an N_2O outlet. Consequently, in attempting to comply with the request, the technician turned the N_2O connector upside down and connected it into the CO_2 outlet instead.

Problem
The N_2O connector is color-coded blue and has notches in the 12 and 5 o'clock positions. The CO_2 connector is color-coded gray and has notches in the 12 and 7 o'clock positions. When the N_2O connector is turned upside down (rotated 180 degrees), it fits into the CO_2 outlet (*see* Figure 8-8, page 132).

Solution
The solution was to design a new N_2O connector that had a peg on the lower edge so that it is impossible to plug it in upside down. The face plate already had a hole in the lower edge to accept the peg, so the only change was to apply the new connector to the N_2O hose (*see* Figure 8-9, page 133). Although the patient was not harmed in this situation, it is alarming to see that color- and shape-coded connectors could still be used incorrectly.

FUTURE DIRECTION FOR HFE AT BJC—AND ELSEWHERE
Improvement projects such as those I have described here not only create a safer environment for employees and patients, they also open up opportunities for more applications of HFE interventions. HFE input is critical to designing new systems, as well as assessing the reliability and robustness of existing systems.

131

Figure 8-8. Nitrogen Oxide (N_2O) and Carbon Dioxide (CO_2) Connectors

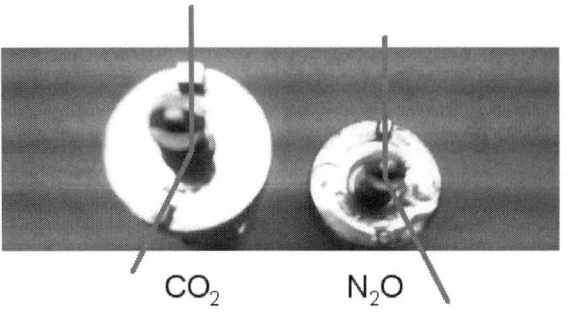
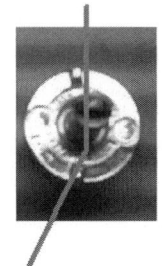

CO₂   N₂O
Notch coding (size and position)

N_2O flipped upside down (180 degrees)

The N_2O and CO_2 connectors are shown at left. When the N_2O connector is turned upside down (rotated 180 degrees), it fits into the CO_2 outlet. The CO_2 connector is color-coded gray and has notches in the 12 and 7 o'clock positions (right). A color version of this figure is also provided online (http://www.jcrinc.com/UHFE10/extras).

Source: BJC HealthCare, St. Louis. Used with permission.

One opportunity to sustain interventions is to attempt to design safety into the hospital environment and equipment. Collaboration with the design and construction department early in the design stage will help to develop standardization and build in safety features. We need to develop evidenced-based practices around design features that will enhance consistent behaviors and promote transparency to reduce confusion and interruptions.

Another area for continuous improvement is to deploy human factors methodology in responding to an adverse event, which can provide broader insights into the system processes involved. Checklists with human factors issues such as sensory perception factors; medical and physiological factors; knowledge/skills, personality, and safety attitudes; and judgment/risk decision factors will help ensure that root cause analyses and Failure Mode and Effects Analyses will be comprehensive.

We plan to incorporate HFE training into patient safety specialists' staff meetings. We will experiment with a checklist that can be used during root cause analysis sessions to promote more comprehensive considerations. Past sessions will be reevaluated to see if any additional causes are generated by the HFE checklist. We will try to develop a "trigger" that will reveal when the specialists should include me in their multidisciplinary evaluations. We also plan to use a structured approach emphasizing Lean Six Sigma tools, HFE concepts, and change management techniques in a project management framework to ensure timely identification and implementation of interventions to prevent recurrences. To structure this approach, we plan to combine strategies currently being employed

CHAPTER 8
Applying Human Factors Engineering in a Patient Safety and Quality Program

Figure 8-9. Old and New Nitrogen Oxide (N$_2$O) Connectors

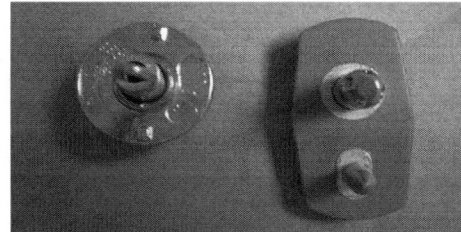
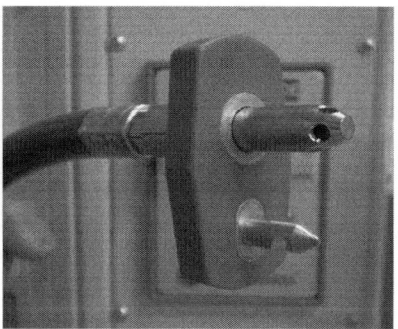

Frontal views of the old and new N$_2$O connectors are shown at left, with a side view of the new N$_2$O connector at right. A color version of this figure is also provided online (http://www.jcrinc.com/UHFE10/ extras).

Source: BJC HealthCare, St. Louis. Used with permission.

in BJC's transformation efforts, including (a) project management; (b) rational process tools[6]; (c) Lean Six Sigma engineering approaches, including human factors engineering; and (d) formal change management techniques. Project management approaches ensure rigorous identification of project goals and adherence to time lines. Rational process tools ensure an organized approach to situational appraisal, problem analysis, and decision making. Lean Six Sigma tools embody industrial engineering principles that seek to reduce waste in processes and systems, while eliminating variability in their performance. Human factors methodology provides a complete system approach to ensure that solutions will meet the capabilities and limitations of the staff, the patients, and the environment. Change management approaches address barriers and facilitators to implementation. By combining these approaches with the traditional tools of health care epidemiology, it is possible to create an efficient, highly structured, yet creative and flexible process by which to develop solutions to safety problems.

The outcomes of this structured approach will culminate in new interventions to prevent similar events from occurring in the future. These interventions will include development of new policies and procedures, simplification of processes, enhanced standardization, checklists, changes in devices or equipment (including adaptive design changes), enhanced safety communication, improvements in teamwork, and additional independent redundancies

Finally, plans also include my greater involvement in review of adverse safety events, which can often be traced to high workload, lack of communication, and habituation to indicators of possible problems. Using HFE methodology will help a team look beyond a training solution and reveal error-proof solutions whenever possible to prevent recurrences.

References

1. Carayon P.: *Handbook of Human Factors and Ergonomics in Health Care and Patient Safety.* Mahwah, NJ: Lawrence-Erlbaum, 2006.
2. George M.L.: *Lean Six Sigma: Combining Six Sigma Quality with Lean Speed.* New York City: McGraw-Hill, 2002.
3. McDermott R.E., Mikulak R.J., Beauregard M.R.: *The Basics of FMEA.* Portland, OR: Productivity, Inc., 1996.
4. Salvendy G.: *Handbook of Human Factors and Ergonomics.* New York City: John Wiley & Sons, Inc., 1997.
5. George M.L., et al.: *The Lean Six Sigma Pocket Toolbook" A Quick Reference Guide to 100 Tools for Improving Quality and Speed.* New York City: McGraw-Hill, 2005.
6. Kepner C.H., Tregoe B.B.: *The New Rational Manager.* Princeton, NJ: Princeton Research Press, 2006.

CHAPTER 9

Integrating Human Factors Engineering Expertise into Patient Safety Research

Yan Xiao, Ph.D.

MY JOURNEY IN HUMAN FACTORS ENGINEERING IN HEALTH CARE

My first venture into health care, in 1989, occurred at the invitation of an anesthesiologist to observe a craniotomy. Although, as an engineer, I did not understand much of what was going on, the visit led me soon after to choose anesthesia as the domain for my doctoral research in human factors. My subsequent three years' experience in field observation and around operating rooms (ORs) taught me two major lessons. First, like an anthropologist conducting field research, one needs to learn about the native "language," customs, aspirations, social norms, and culture. In the case of anesthesia, it was important to learn work routines to remember basic terminologies and principles of pharmacology and physiology and to appreciate the social milieu of the OR. Second, as an outsider, one has to be humble, to listen and learn what the "natives" describe as their problems. My initial problem statement for my doctoral research was how to display patient physiologic parameters to best support anesthesiologists' ability to diagnose problems and manage crises during surgery. Through observation and conversation with anesthesiologists of different training levels, I gradually learned to appreciate the key problem-solving strategies that anesthesiologists use to ensure patient safety. For example, experienced anesthesiologists, in preparing for surgery, anticipate potential problems and rehearse possible solutions,[1] taking care to stock the workspace with specially needed supplies and medication. The functional roles of such planning activities are very similar to those uncovered in studies of planning of fighter-plane pilots.

In the 1990s I was fortunate to know some of the leaders in patient safety in anesthesia, such as David Gaba, Jeff Cooper, and Matt Weinger. They showed me case examples of the human factors contribution to patient safety, as seen, for example, in the fail-safe design of vaporizers in anesthesia machines, studies of the deleterious effects of fatigue on vigilance, and simulation-based crew resource management. Also, I remember the wall panel of lookalike ampoules on display in the anesthesia lounge of the Toronto General to remind anesthesiologists of the danger of picking up unintended drugs.

At the University of Maryland School of Medicine, one of the first medical schools to hire human factors engineers or other human factors engineering (HFE) professionals as faculty members, I quickly became involved in a wide variety of HFE research, as reflected in the following projects:

> ### Figure 9-1. Views of Thoracostomy Instrument Trays
>
>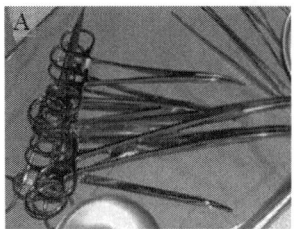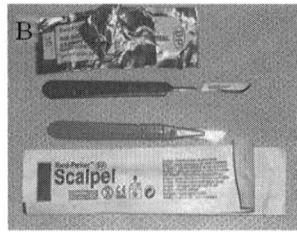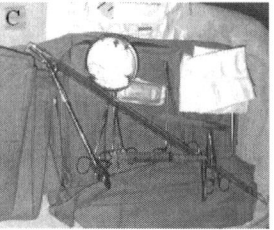
>
> Views of the original thoracostomy instrument tray are provided: (A) constellation of instruments threaded on a needle driver; (B) reusable scalpel handle with disposable blade (top), and disposable scalpel (bottom); (C) the newly designed thoracostomy instrument tray when fully prepped, showing thoracostomy tube, anesthetic syringe, and disposable scalpel.
>
> **Source:** Seagull F.J., et al.: Video-based ergonomic analysis to evaluate thoracostomy tube placement techniques. *J Trauma* 60:227–232, Jan. 2006. Used with permission.

- Video-clip ergonomic analysis of thoracostomy (for relief of pneumo- or hemothorax) techniques to identify risks to the patient and operator, including instrument-tray positioning and instrument content[2] (*see* Figure 9-1, above). Video analysis of central line and chest tube placement revealed several ways in which sterile fields were contaminated
- Video clips from actual line placement also provide powerful training materials to engage trainees and to learn about what *not* do through detailed task analysis.[3]
- Interviews of team members at a trauma resuscitation unit led to an understanding of the team leadership's need to balance training and patient care, so that attending surgeons and fellows sometimes ceded control of patient care to the less experienced members of the team.[4]
- Observations of "artifacts" used by OR teams uncovered a sophisticated sociotechnical system for coordinating the flow of personnel, patients, and instruments. Computer-supported cooperative work-design principles were used in developing technology enhancements. For example, careful design and detailed interview studies led to implementation of sensitive video technology to augment the manual OR whiteboard.[5]
- Videotaping of rounding in pediatric intensive care units revealed the inefficiency of communication. Adoption of available tools and changes in rounding, such as the structure of case presentations, were recommended to shorten data retrieval and presentation time to the benefit of discussion and teaching.[6]
- Interviews and observations suggested that the problem of "failure to respond" to auditory alarms reflected the large numbers of alarms, confusion of alarms, temporary episodes of high workload, and external economic pressures. Instead of engaging in an "arms race" for attention with louder and more disruptive alarms, efforts should be made to reduce the overall number of alarms and to make judicious use of monitored beds, which produce alarm events based on patient monitors.[7]
- A systems engineering approach, which

includes but goes beyond HFE, is often needed to embrace the variety of expertise needed to solve a given problem. For example, in the case of the OR work flow, contributing factors included deficiencies in the design of the built environment, communication among staff, and scheduling techniques.[5] In one surgical suite, only one elevator was big enough for transporting cardiac patients with attached monitors and devices, but three cardiac cases were to start at the same time in the morning. Thus, expertise in process modeling and architecture was needed to appreciate the problem. Operations research provides techniques to use simulation to understand the impact of different scheduling practices.

In 2009, after spending 15 years of academic research in patient safety and working with hospitals to improve patient safety, I changed careers to work for the Baylor Health Care System (Dallas) as the system director for patient safety research. In this role, I lead the department in its efforts to (1) undertake multidisciplinary investigations, building on existing research in place in the Office of Patient Safety and collaborating with outside researchers in health care and related fields such as engineering; (2) improve fundamental understanding of safe health care delivery and contribute to the evidence base of patient safety improvement strategies; and (3) provide guidance for the long-term direction of patient safety at Baylor. The position is funded by a combination of system operations and internal projects and extramural projects.

APPLYING HFE IN PATIENT SAFETY AT BAYLOR HEALTH CARE SYSTEM
Infrastructure

The Department of Patient Safety Research is housed within the corporate Office of Patient Safety and is also a member division of the corporate research arm, the Institute for Health Care Research and Improvement; I report to the vice president for patient safety. The department has a full-time health services researcher and two full-time nurses, who, as patient safety champions, coordinate the implementation of patient safety intiatives (such as the current World Health Organization's Surgical Safety Checklist).

Collaboration is undertaken with physicians and other clinicians and staff at other entities within the Baylor Health System (such as nursing research and education, health care improvement, and information technology), and with other institutions in the Dallas area to use its inpatient and ambulatory care settings as a "laboratory." Over time, collaboration should also occur with university laboratories (for example, for innovation in tool development, as associated with medical informatics and training).

Recruitment and Roles of HFE Professionals

Recruitment. Planning is under way to add more positions for HFE professionals who can work with clinicians to find innovative ways to reduce the risk of patient harm and to increase the efficiency and quality of frontline staff's work lives.

Given the wide range of HFE professionals' education and training, as discussed in Chapter 4, as well as the wide spectrum of health care issues and problems in need of HFE expertise, health care organizations should be flexible when identifying the most appropriate candidates. It is unrealistic to expect a newly hired HFE professional to be able to immediately start work on the "problem of the day." Organizations should be prepared to provide additional training in terms of both human factors subspecialty areas and skills, such as usability and team performance, and exposure to different settings, ranging from a primary care practice to the OR. Yet all

HFE professionals should be conversant with the benefits and risks associated with information technology, given its increasingly central role in health care delivery.

Roles. Organizationally, HFE professionals should be prepared to function as educators and project consultants, often for clinical effectiveness or quality improvement teams. Nurses and other clinicians may first learn about the field of HFE and its concepts and methods in the course of collaborating with the HFE professional. They might then learn more specific applications, such as safety through design and limitations of human vigilance, either in further personal interaction or in workshops and internal or external courses (*see* Chapters 6 and 8). Incremental courses and educational materials, in development on an ongoing basis, are used to promote the HFE skill sets of frontline staff, who would then be in a position to apply their learning to their everyday work. HFE professionals, who usually have been trained in taxonomies of human errors, can provide human factors expertise in root cause analysis (RCA) for risk managers and other RCA team members, helping the team to develop solutions that are likely to succeed in the long term. HFE professionals can also guide rapid prototyping by assessing different solutions through cognitive walk-throughs and other techniques.

The education campaign to promote frontline staff's HFE skills sets has already been reflected in the implementation teams' requests for consultation and information to help them with their specific design projects. For example, for a project on the choice of hardware for bedside computers, the team was advised to develop specific scenarios, such as patient education and shift sign-out, and then involve nurses and other users to help anticipate potential problems. The project team had planned to organize focus groups with little structure, more along the lines of building user buy-in as opposed to assessing usability. Such scenario-based evaluation methodologies were likely to work well with the planned mock-up stations. In carrying out the potential usage scenarios, the teams were taught how to identify the respective effects of different options of bedside monitors on work flow, staff interactions, and staff-patient interactions. At the onset of the project, I introduced human factors in terms of physical ergonomics—for example, whether the height of the computer monitors needed to be adjustable. By thinking through concrete-usage scenarios, nurses quickly identified the key issues when attempting to incorporate bedside computer monitors into their work flow.

After the type of bedside computer monitor is chosen, it is anticipated that the monitors, when installed, will be used to show education materials directly to patients and family members. The nurses on the implementation teams quickly realized the need to coach patients and families to navigate the computer screens so that they could then interact with the computers directly.

HFE professionals should be involved in or even lead projects when the focus is on design or acquisition activities. For example, in implementation teams for health information technology, the HFE professional with expertise in human-computer interaction can lead Failure Mode and Effects Analysis sessions on computerized order entry and clinical decision support systems. Typically, the implementation teams, which are charged with the responsibilities of designing, ordering, and charting screens, include pharmacy, nursing, and physician users as clinical subject matter experts. Human factors–related issues, such as user-error predictions, training needs, screen layout, and clinical alerts, come up frequently. As project lead, the HFE professional can bring in subject matter

CHAPTER 9
Integrating Human Factors Engineering Expertise into Patient Safety Research

experts, organize user-requirement analysis, and develop plans to assess usability. For acquisition teams, the HFE professional, who may be a member of a biomedical engineering department,* can lead in technology assessment, developing evaluation metrics and requests for proposals, and conducting usability testing.

Two of the initial areas of focus at Baylor Health Care System were implementing electronic health record (EHR) systems and enhancing patient education for self-care skills.

Case Study 1. Implementation of Electronic Health Records

In an ongoing project on the improvement of safety associated with the implementation of EHRs at the Baylor Health Care System, my role has been a combination of educator and internal consultant. As educator, I have conducted one-on-one meetings with key stakeholders to assess the need for education regarding the potential contributions of HFE, provided short presentations on an overview of human factors to executive teams, and synthesized summaries of research findings on medical informatics and human factors. Staff were told that as an internal consultant, I would provide advice on hazards analysis and on the building of EHR screens. The importance of human factors to safety in EHRs has not always been intuitive to key decision makers, a situation I addressed with a written communication, as shown in Sidebar 9-1 (page 140), to key stakeholders.

Unanticipated Consequences of EHR. Human factors principles were used to synthesize and interpret published reports on the so-called unanticipated consequences of EHR. For example, the following list was used to communicate about the potential risks of current screen design:
- Overly cluttered screen design
- Poor use of available screen space
- Inconsistencies in screen design
- Lists not easily sorted
- Screens hard to read or annotate
- Minimum availability of defaults
- Lack of appropriate safeguards to prevent selecting the wrong patient or entering incorrect data

Because of such design flaws, EHRs may induce hazards to care delivery. Again, the literature was used to illustrate occurrences of "user errors" that should be anticipated, such as the following:
- Selecting a patient name adjacent to the intended name
- Making a wrong selection in long, dense pick lists
- Missing critical laboratory results buried multiple clicks away
- Clicking through alert screens with low specific clinical value

The current literature is an important source of HFE theory and examples. For example, a recent study of the use of root cause analysis of patient misidentification in laboratory medicine showed that the incorrect selection of menu items was a leading cause of patient misidentification.[8] Of 132 misidentification events occurring in the preanalytic testing phase, wrist bands labeled for the wrong patient were applied on admission ($n = 8$), and laboratory tests were ordered for the wrong patient by selecting the wrong electronic medical record from a menu of similar names and Social Security numbers ($n = 31$).

---

* Several engineering fields, such as biomedical engineering, have traditionally been part of a hospital's workforce. Because these fields share some of the training with HFE, one option is to embed human factors engineers within the departments that traditionally hire other engineers.

> ### Sidebar 9-1. Communication on Human Factors Engineering and Electronic Health Records
>
> Research on the impact of electronic health record (EHR) systems has provided insights into new types of errors and thus risks to patients ("e-iatrogenesis"). There have been published reports on potential harm of poor implementation of EHRs, including one study that associated the implementation of a computerized order entry system in a teaching hospital to increased mortality (6.8% from 2.8%).[1] Reported error types facilitated by EHRs include entering orders on the wrong patient, nurses not knowing an order had been generated, desensitization to alerts, wrong medication dosing, and overlapping medication orders.[2] Human factors engineering (HFE) has been advocated to fit technologies to organizational, team, and individual needs.[3] HFE can also contribute to meet several "grand challenges" in clinical decision support,[4] such as improving the human-computer interface, summarizing patient-level information, and prioritizing recommendations to the user.
>
> **References**
> 1. Han Y.Y., et al.: Unexpected increased mortality after implementation of a commercially sold computerized physician order entry system. *Pediatrics* 116:1506–1512, Dec. 2005.
> 2. Campbell E.M., et al.: Types of unintended consequences related to computerized provider order entry. *J Am Med Inform Assoc* 13:547–556, Sep.–Oct. 2006.
> 3. Walker J.M., et al.: EHR safety: The way forward to safe and effective systems. *J Am Med Inform Assoc* 15:272–277, May–Jun. 2008. Epub Feb. 28, 2008.
> 4. Sittig D.F., et al. Grand challenges in clinical decision support. *J Biomed Inform* 41:387–392, Apr. 2008.
>
> **Source:** Baylor Health Care System, Dallas. Used with permission.

Through the EHR project Baylor is in the process of institutionalizing the involvement of HFE professionals, as in the following:
1. Training and education of design teams in principles of usability and human factors as related to EHR
2. Inclusion of usability expertise in design and assessment
3. Usability testing as part of design cycles
4. Mechanisms for continuous usability monitoring and improvement

Hazard analysis was used in the EHR project to examine potential harm caused by shortcomings, among other factors, in human-computer interactions (for example, data hidden in pages, therefore difficult to navigate to), disruptions of staff communication patterns (misleading task status indicators), and "brittle" automation (automated work flow for medication orders that relies on timely human data entry). The procedures to carry out hazard analysis were as follows:
1. Cognitive task analysis of information needs and potential data overload through qualitative methods
2. Development of metrics for monitoring EHR safety through automatically captured usage logs
3. Development of checklists for identifying hazards in EHR interfaces, EHR–associated work-flow changes, and EHR–induced changes in communication

As one of the tangible outcomes of the hazard analysis, resources were set aside for engaging human factors experts in developing strategies to reduce hazards associated with the work-flow changes.

Illustration of Potential Errors. When working with screen-design teams, I used examples of existing screen designs to illustrate potential errors on the basis of human factors principles. For example, one principle is that working memory, as a very limited resource and very vulnerable to interruptions, should be supported. Pop-up screens to solicit input from users are frequent, thereby blocking off key vital information about the patient, such as medical record number, body weight, location, and allergies. Although users may see such vital information while viewing the primary screen, they may not retain the accurate information in working memory and may be interrupted for other tasks. Therefore, pop-up screens should contain the information needed for accomplishing the task at hand without relying on the users' ability to retain accurate information in the working memory.

Given the HFE principle that visual search is often sequential but nonsystematic, screen organization should facilitate visual scanning. Busy screens in the existing EHR design were used to illustrate poor visual alignment, which make it difficult for users to hunt and find the information needed. I suggested grouping information by inserting visual boundaries and by aligning items.

On-the-Job Education of the Teams. In my experience, EHR design team members are usually aware of some HFE–related issues, such as those concerning human-computer interface (as in font selection). However, their knowledge about cognitive and perceptual limitations, as in working memory and visual scanning, is often inadequate. Team members are often guided by "folk models" of human cognition, which assume, for example, flawless working memory. I used my interactions with the design teams, such as when considering specific screen designs, as an opportunity to explain broader HFE principles.

Another ongoing project is to improve education of patient self-care skills, as described in the next case study.

Case Study 2. Education of Patient Self-Care Skills

Health care organizations are increasingly held accountable for patient outcomes, ranging from across episodes of care, from hospitalization to postdischarge. In the case of congestive heart failure (CHF), for example, although compliance with evidence-based guidelines for inpatient care has increased dramatically over the last decade, the 30-day mortality and rehospitalization rates of patients have been persistently high across the United States.[9,10]

An assessment of current practices at Baylor demonstrated wide variability in patient education. Many patient education activities were delivered through handouts of printed materials—which have been shown, however, to be ineffective.[11,12]

It is not well known that HFE principles and methods can be used to address patient motivation, self-care expertise development, and educational techniques.[13] To expand HFE awareness at Baylor, we initiated an expertise-study project in preparation of interventions to disseminate best practices. We assembled a project team (composed of a human factors specialist, a nurse manager, a health services researcher, two heart-failure-clinic nurses, and a hospitalist) to conduct a cognitive task analysis project to elicit the practices used by the expert team in a nurse-led heart-failure clinic who have been able to achieve low readmission rates for CHF patients. We conducted informal-knowledge elicitation sessions on the basis of the principles of cognitive task analysis.[14] For example, one of the techniques used in eliciting expertise is to focus on experts' own assessment of what makes a task difficult and the types of errors a nonexpert would be likely to commit. The leading expert in the clinical team—a nurse who is also a member of the project team—discussed a series of recent interactions with patients concerning postdischarge plans, in which she identified barriers in self-care (such as lack of skills to monitor symptoms) and then focused on helping the patient develop problem-solving skills to address them. She pointed out common mistakes in patient education, such as lack of engagement with the patients and a lack of individualization of problem solving.

The anticipated project deliverables will include detailed tactics and training scenarios for wider adoption. Tactics might include, for example, rapid diagnosis of deficits in patient self-care skills and methods to use patients' own words to link symptoms with underlying disease processes.

Of course, the reduction of readmission rates depends on many additional factors, such as access to primary care and coordination of care across settings. Like many problems in health care, preventing readmissions requires an integrated approach that includes multiple components, such as care coordination for access to primary care, community resources and new care delivery models with multitier care providers. The current interest in "medical home" provides more opportunities for human factors engineers to help with design care delivery systems and with ways to improve care coordination. Although the dominant portion of research efforts has been on developing interventions and on evaluating efficacy of interventions, how to translate evidence into effective care delivery systems provides a strong impetus for human factors engineers.

CONCLUSION

Since the Institute of Medicine's *To Err Is Human* report,[15] which cited an HFE–based principle, "Respect Human Limits In Process Design," HFE has become increasingly deployed in improving patient safety. However, to my knowledge, relatively few health care organizations are known to have instituted formal human factors programs and hired full-time HFE professionals. A number of barriers exist to fully capitalize on the expertise of human factors engineers in health care delivery systems, not the least of which is the infrequent communication between HFE and health care providers. Baylor started to address this barrier by incrementally educating clinical and administrative leadership about human factors. The ongoing project on EHR implementation (Case Study 1) is being used as a prototype of how HFE can be used to improve patient safety.

Given the wide range of human factors issues, and the correspondingly large potential of contributions from HFE, there may not be a single best way of using human factors expertise and developing a comprehensive portfolio of human factors activities. Rather, each health care organization should prioritize its own patient safety areas, be they in team communications, implementation of EHR, or medical devices, and proceed from there.

CHAPTER 9
Integrating Human Factors Engineering Expertise into Patient Safety Research

References

1. Xiao Y., Milgram P., Doyle D.J.: Planning behavior and its functional role in the interaction with complex systems. *IEEE Transactions on Systems, Man, and Cybernetics, Part A: Systems and Humans* 27:313–324, May 1997.
2. Seagull F.J., et al.: Video-based ergonomic analysis to evaluate thoracostomy tube placement techniques. *J Trauma* 60:227–232, Jan. 2006.
3. Xiao Y., et al.: Video-based training increases sterile-technique compliance during central venous catheter insertion. *Crit Care Med* 35:1302–1306, May 2007.
4. Klein K., et al.: Dynamic delegation: Shared, hierarchical, deindividualized leadership in extreme action teams. *Administrative Science Quarterly* 51(4):590–621, 2006.
5. Xiao Y., et al.: Opportunities and challenges in improving surgical work flow. *Cognition, Technology & Work* 10:313–321, Oct. 2008.
6. Cardarelli M., et al.: Dissecting multidisciplinary cardiac surgery rounds. *Ann Thorac Surg* 88:809–813, Sep. 2009.
7. Xiao Y., et al.: Organizational-historical analysis of the "failure to respond to alarm" problem. *IEEE Transactions on Systems, Man, and Cybernetics, Part A: Systems and Humans* 34:772–778, Nov. 2004.
8. Dunn E.J., Moga P.J. Patient misidentification in laboratory medicine: A qualitative analysis of 227 root cause analysis reports in the Veterans Health Administration. *Arch Pathol Lab Med* 134:244–255, Feb. 2010.
9. Gwadry-Sridhar F.H., et al.: A systematic review and meta-analysis of studies comparing readmission rates and mortality rates in patients with heart failure. *Arch Intern Med* 164:2315–2320, Nov. 22, 2004.
10. O'Connell J.B:. The economic burden of heart failure. *Clin Cardiol* 23(3 suppl.):III6–III10, Mar. 2000.
11. Moser D.K., Doering L.V., Chung M.L.: Vulnerabilities of patients recovering from an exacerbation of chronic heart failure. *Am Heart J* 150:984, Nov. 2005.
12. Dickson V.V., Riegel B.: Are we teaching what patients need to know? Building skills in heart failure self-care. *Heart Lung* 38:253–261, May–Jun. 2009, Epub Jan. 21, 2009.
13. Lippa K.D., Klein H.A., Shalin V.L.: Everyday expertise: Cognitive demands in diabetes self-management. *Hum Factors* 50:112–120, Feb. 2008.
14. Klein G.A., Calderwood R., MacGregor D.: Critical decision method for eliciting knowledge. *IEEE Trans Syst Man Cybern* 19(3):462–472, May-Jun., 1989.
15. Institute of Medicine: *To Err Is Human: Building a Safer Health System.* Washington, DC: National Academy Press, 1999.

CHAPTER 10

Integrating Human Factors Engineering into Medication Safety at ISMP Canada

Sylvia Hyland, R.Ph., B.Sc.Phm., M.H.Sc.; John Senders, Ph.D.

BACKGROUND AND SCOPE OF WORK AT ISMP CANADA

The Institute for Safe Medication Practices Canada (ISMP Canada),[1] a sister organization to ISMP in the United States,[2] was created in 2000 with the mandate to analyze medication incidents (an alternative term for medication errors), and make recommendations for medication system improvements. ISMP Canada began as a team of five founding members, joined by an intensive care unit (ICU) pharmacist with an interest in information technology, who believed that patient safety was important and that poorly designed systems facilitate mistakes by practitioners.

During the early days, the members of the initial staff team worked in health care organizations whose leaders were supportive of ISMP Canada's efforts. A decade after its formation, ISMP Canada is widely recognized as a resource for analyzing information about medication incidents in Canada and has collaborative relations with a range of strategic partners, at the provincial, national, and international levels. For example, ISMP Canada worked with Health Canada and the Canadian Institute for Health Information (http://secure.cihi.ca/cihiweb/splash.html) to develop the Canadian Medication Incident Reporting and Prevention System.*[3] Reports of medication incidents from practitioners and consumers are received by ISMP Canada through a variety of channels, including Web portal and phone. Although the reporting of medication incidents is voluntary, and despite the unavailability of denominator information such as drug usage data for error-probability calculations, we do know that multiple reports about a specific product or procedure typically signify an issue worth investigating. At times, even one report serves as a flag for the entire health care system of an unacceptable risk requiring analysis of the underlying causes.

---

* *Medication incident:* Any preventable event that may cause or lead to inappropriate medication use or patient harm while the medication is in the control of the health care professional, patient, or consumer. Medication incidents may be related to professional practice, drug products, procedures, and systems, and include prescribing, order communication, product labeling/packaging/ nomenclature, compounding, dispensing, distribution, administration, education, monitoring, and use.
Source: ISMP Canada: *Definition of Terms.* http://www.ismp-canada.org/definitions.htm (accessed May 6, 2010).

Medication errors that result in harm attract the greatest attention in the news media; however, ISMP Canada accepts and analyzes data on errors whether or not they result in harm, including errors that were caught or corrected. We believe that every error can provide important information in terms of how the system presented an opportunity for it to occur. Thus, ISMP Canada operates under the principle that if we are to understand medication errors, it is important to capture information on all of them.

ROLE OF HUMAN FACTORS ENGINEERING IN MEDICATION SAFETY

ISMP Canada recognized early on that its core competencies required more than the expertise of pharmacists, nurses, physicians, and administrators—they also depended on the insights derived from human factors engineering (HFE). To err may be human, but errors in health care are often rooted in problems of system design. The true value of HFE quickly became apparent as the organization began to tackle real-world problems, such as an early project on sterile water (Case Study 3). One of the founding members [J.S.], who has expertise in psychology, law, and engineering, introduced the principles of HFE to ISMP Canada as a key component of systems thinking and incident analysis and system redesign solutions. Michael Cohen (ISMP in the United States), another founding member, introduced the group to an HFE consultant (John Gosbee), who subsequently assisted with staff training and provided the fundamentals of heuristic evaluation, usability testing, and other human factors concepts.

HFE can be used to improve people's ability to catch their own errors and the errors of others—and to preventing them from happening in the first place. To avoid a "culture of blame,"

one must focus on (1) the human factors as well as the environmental/system factors that contributed to the incident and (2) the opportunities for reducing both the probability of a similar incident and the probability that such an incident will injure a patient. We now present case studies to illustrate the use of HFE in medication safety.

Case Study 1. Fentanyl Transdermal Patches

Fentanyl transdermal patches are designed to manage persistent, moderate-to-severe chronic pain in opioid-tolerant patients by releasing an opioid medication at a constant rate to be absorbed through the skin. The patches provide a controlled-release dose, an easy-to-administer option when patients cannot be managed by other means such as oral opioid products. ISMP Canada received reports of concern from physicians when one of the patch products was introduced to the Canadian market. Practitioners in emergency departments had failed to see the patches on patients. Figure 10-1a (page 147) shows a fentanyl patch as it appears after being removed from its backing.

Because it was almost invisible, health care providers, as well as care providers in the home, had no visible sign to make them aware that a patch was in place. Invisible patches were a particular problem when there was a transition for patients, such as coming to an emergency department (ED), transferring from the ED to an inpatient unit, or transferring from an acute care hospital to a long term care facility.

The HFE solution to this problem was relatively simple—give the patch some color that distinguishes it from the skin and provide the drug name and dose, as shown in Figure 10-1b (page 147). Not only is the patch now visible but important safety information for the prescriber and the patient is also displayed.

Figure 10-1. Fentanyl Patch: After Removal from Backing and After Problem Solved

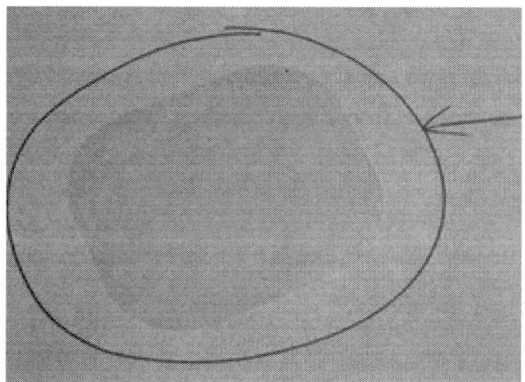
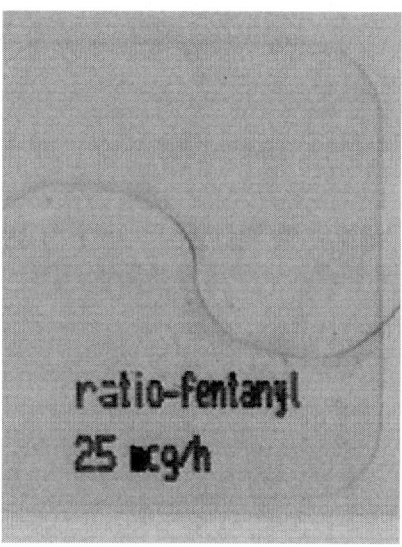

Figure 10-1a (left) shows a fentanyl patch (circled) as it appears after being removed from its backing. The HFE solution to this problem was to give the patch some color that distinguishes it from the skin and provide identification with the drug name and dose (Figure 10-1b, right). A color version of this figure is also provided online (http:/www.jcrinc.com/UHFE10/extras).

Source: ISMP Canada. Used with permission.

Case Study 2. Calcium Gluconate

Product packaging can play an important role in medication incidents, and sometimes even small changes can increase safety. Figure 10-2a (page 148) shows a vial of calcium gluconate as it was originally labeled. Note that the drug concentration is given in molar units of millimoles (mmol) per 10 milliliter (mL, a measure of volume).

However, although the labeling met the needs of pharmacists and hospital pharmacy technicians who prepared total parenteral nutrition solutions, it confused physicians and nurses working in patient care areas. Physicians pre-scribe calcium gluconate in weight units of grams (g) or milligrams (mg). Therefore, when a physician prescribed calcium gluconate, the nurse would need to convert grams to mmol to calculate how much to withdraw from the vial. Each added step to the process of medication administration is an added opportunity for error that can be difficult to detect before it reaches the patient.

HFE stresses that systems need to be designed to reduce opportunities for errors. For some complex machines, such as electronic infusion pumps, this could mean a design that limits the maximum programmable infusion rate to

Figure 10-2. A Vial of Calcium Gluconate, Before and After

a.

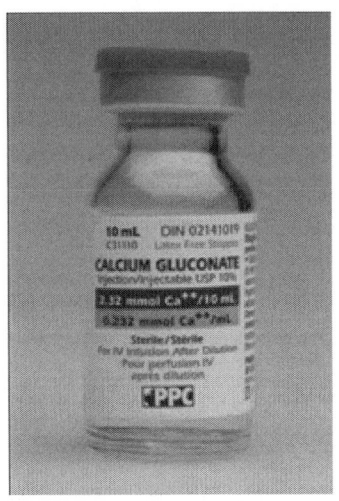

b.

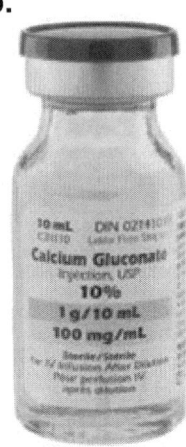

As shown in Figure 10-2a (left), a vial of calcium gluconate, as it was originally labeled, provides the drug concentration in molar units of millimoles (mmol) per 10 milliliter (mL, a measure of volume). In the revised package label, the concentration is now expressed in grams per total volume and milligrams per mL (Figure 10-2b, right). A color version of this figure is also provided online (http:/www.jcrinc.com/UHFE10/extras).

Source: ISMP Canada. Used with permission.

---

prevent catastrophic errors. In the case of calcium gluconate, it would have made complex calculations, in a patient care area, unnecessary.

Figure 10-2b (above) shows the revised package label, with the concentration now expressed in grams per total volume and milligrams per mL. (The drug concentration in molar units of millimoles (mmol) per milliliter, useful information for pharmacy compounding, is provided on the side panel of the vial label). In addition, the manufacturer went further and demonstrated leadership in safety by removing the company logo to provide space for, and give prominence to the critical information on the front panel of the label.

Case Study 3. Sterile Water

ISMP Canada has released bulletins warning abut the potential for harm resulting from intravenous (IV) administration of sterile water.[4,5] Sterile water is used to dilute certain medications for injection but should not itself be directly infused intravenously. It is hypotonic and can cause hemolysis, which can lead to renal complications and serious patient harm.

Sterile water is marketed in a flexible bag very similar to those used for IV solutions (*see* Figure 10-3a, page 149). It is easy for someone to pick up the wrong bag.

CHAPTER 10
Integrating Human Factors Engineering into Medication Safety at ISMP Canada

> **Figure 10-3. Labeling for Sterile Water for Injection, Before and After, in Comparison with Intravenous (IV) Solutions**
>
> a.
>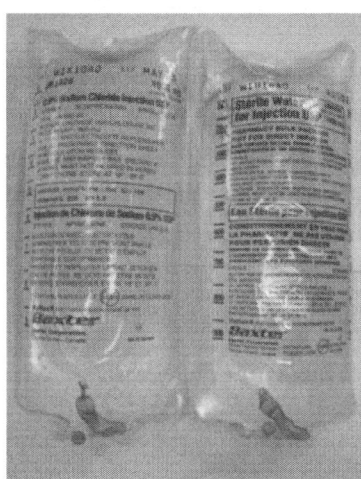
>
> b.
>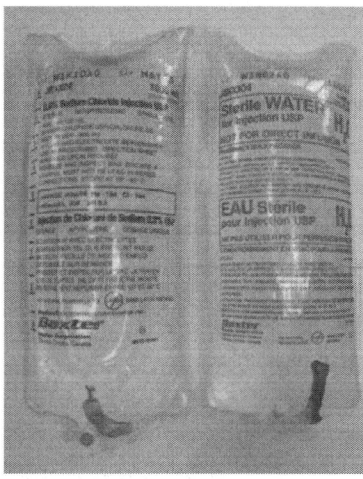
>
> As shown in Figure 10-3a, an IV solution—0.9% sodium chloride injection—and the former sterile water for injection product (on the right side) both had labels with black print. The new label for sterile water for injection product (on the right side) combines color, information display, and redundant cues to help differentiate the product from IV solutions. A color version of this figure is also provided online (http:/www.jcrinc.com/UHFE10/extras).
>
> **Source:** ISMP Canada. Used with permission.

In this case, changing the entire packaging was not feasible because of manufacturing limitations. Instead, ISMP Canada worked with the product manufacturer to design label improvements that would enhance patient safety yet were within the capacity of their manufacturing equipment. The label improvements were as follows and are shown in Figure 10-3b (above):

- *The use of color:* The color of the print on the label was changed from all black to all red to send a message of warning to those handling the bags and to differentiate the label from regular IV solutions.
- *Making critical information prominent:* The words "not for direct infusion" were given prominence on the new label. In addition, varied font size ("water" is in large uppercase letters) and the use of varied upper- and lowercase lettering help distinguish information. The official United States Pharmacopeia (USP) name *Sterile Water for Injection* can mislead health care practitioners to think it appropriate to administer intravenously. Because the official USP name is a requirement, the new label deemphasizes the words "for injection" by printing them in smaller size and in lower-case lettering.
- *Use of redundant cues*: Using the international chemical H_2O symbol adds a "redundant cue" to the label, helping users to identify the product as water. The use of multiple

redundant cues (for example, unique container shape and material) would further assist users in differentiating between similarly packaged products.

It was particularly rewarding to see that the competing manufacturer also changed its labeling of sterile water in a similar manner. Our hope and challenge is that the learning from incidents and resultant label improvements is not lost over time. How do we ensure organizational and health care system memory? One opportunity currently planned is to work with regulators and provide input to new labeling guidelines that incorporate a requirement for evidence-based enhanced labeling for safety.

Using Failure Mode and Effects Analysis

An important part of the process for recommending the changes to the product label design for packaging of the sterile-water product was the testing of the changes using Failure Mode and Effects Analysis (FMEA). FMEA is a proactive safety technique that is used to help identify process and product problems before they occur—an important consideration when making recommendations or implementing change. Widely used in improving quality and safety in industry (for example, the automotive, aviation, and nuclear power industries), it can be applied to a wide range of health care processes, including medication use and medication labeling.

In conducting FMEA, one asks, "What could fail and in what manner?"; "Given the various possibilities for failure, what are the potential consequences of each?"; and "How can harmful consequences be prevented?" The goal is to identify those elements of a system whose failure in specific ways poses a threat to patient safety, as well as those that not only contribute to errors but can be manipulated and used to help detect and reduce errors or to reduce their consequences.[6] ISMP Canada follows eight critical steps in its FMEAs:

1. Select a process to analyze and assemble an appropriate team.
2. Diagram the process, break it into its elemental parts, and perform a cognitive walk-through.
3. Identify potential failure modes of each part and determine their effects.
4. Identify the causes of failure modes.
5. Prioritize failure modes.
6. Redesign the components, as well as the whole process, as needed.
7. Analyze and test the changes.
8. Implement and monitor the redesigned process.

In other words, the goal is to identify actions, elements, or processes that can cause errors; their underlying causes; and opportunities for improvement.[7] The next case study describes a project in which components of an FMEA, rather than a full FMEA, were used to identify and evaluate opportunities for medication system improvement.

Case Study 4. Emergency Medical Service Medication Kit

In this project we applied HFE to medication safety in prehospital care, with a focus on a medication kit used in emergency medical services (EMS). The kit was created as part of a new protocol, Vital Heart Response (VHR), which was implemented by Edmonton (Alberta) EMS for managing patients experiencing an ST-segment elevation myocardial infarction (STEMI). Soon after implementation of the new protocol in spring 2006, two nonfatal incidents occurred in which the wrong drug was administered. This prompted the VHR development team (members from the Capital Health Region [now a part of Alberta Health Services] and Edmonton EMS) to review the medication kit. The team proposed changes to the medication kit and contracted with ISMP Canada to review and analyze the proposed changes.

The ISMP Canada team lead worked with an HFE consultant to conduct an analysis of the medication kit. The project began with the examination of pictures of the kit (original and proposed design changes) and conducting a preliminary human factors analysis. In addition to examining the physical attributes of the medication kit and its contents, we also needed to understand the context in which it was used. The team lead and HFE consultant visited the VHR team, which had created the protocol, and conducted "knowledge elicitation" with four domain experts and project team members from Edmonton EMS and Alberta Health Services. The team lead and HFE consultant reviewed the VHR protocol and medication kit in detail and viewed their location in the ambulance. It was important to develop an understanding of the communication patterns, information needs, decision-making points, and information flow between the patient, EMS crew, VHR physician, and dispatcher. Attention was focused on the paper forms and the medication kit, which represented a significant portion of the VHR protocol, because their design and ease of use has a direct impact on crew performance and protocol compliance.

The Edmonton EMS managed a STEMI only once or twice a year. The infrequent practice, as well as the lack of a rehearsal policy, would amplify any usability issues and lead to loss of the knowledge gained through training. This made it imperative that the medication kit and associated paper forms be easy to use and easy to translate into actions (including medication selection, preparation, and administration).

Cognitive Walk-through
HFE provided a way to analyze the "ease of use" systematically. One activity that is central to conducting a thorough human factors analysis is the observing of typical usage by a representative user. A cognitive walk-through was conducted by observing an emergency medical technologist-paramedic (EMT-P or paramedic) as he used the forms and medication kit. The participating paramedic last had an encounter with a STEMI patient about six months earlier. It was important to work with an end user who had not had a recent encounter with actual practice so that issues with usability were not masked by recent practice or rehearsal. It was also important that this paramedic not be a member of the team developing the kit and paper forms so that his knowledge of the material would not be biased and would be more representative of that of typical end users.

To conduct the cognitive walk-through, the VHR team created a scenario in which the paramedic participant was responding to a call for a patient complaining of chest pain. We then asked the participant to think out loud as he simulated the steps and activities that he would normally perform in such a call.

This cognitive walk-through yielded valuable information about context of use and the physical and mental activities that led up to the point in which the paper forms and medication kit are retrieved for use. It was possible to establish the high level of workload experienced by the paramedic(s) as they conducted multiple concurrent tasks: coordinating a variety of activities, people and materials; gathering information from the patient; and interacting with a physician (via dispatching system) to establish a diagnosis.

Matching the Protocol to Actual Work Flow
After retrieving the kit, the paramedic followed the protocol explained in the paper forms. Several instances where he needed to shift his focus elsewhere, usually to another page, or to

communicate with the patient to obtain information (for instance, querying the patient), or act on the information obtained (find the "patient consent" form) were identified. The shifting of attention and subsequent return to the protocol involves mental effort. One of our recommendations was a redesign of the paper forms to minimize the need for shifting attention back and forth. Another design recommendation was to embed visual cues to help the paramedic keep track of where he or she left off in the protocol if a shifting of attention is necessary. This is particularly important for work conditions that are characterized by interruptions and multitasking.

Matching the Medication Kit Layout to Protocol Instructions

It was observed that the original kit was designed with primarily text instructions regarding the selection and retrieval of medication. There are several combinations of medications that need to be used in varying doses, depending on the patient's age and type of treatment selected by the physician. The user had to remember this information while orienting himself or herself to the kit and to the organization of the medications. This retrieval process was inefficient and could be improved by providing graphical information in the instructions that were mapped directly to the layout of the kit. In other words, the physical layout of the medications in the VHR medication kit would be reflected in the instructions (*see* Figure 10-4, at right).

Iterative Design

The approach that the VHR team adopted in redesigning its medication kit is one that is central to any human factors project—iterative design. Simply put, iterative design involves conducting human factors analyses or usability tests, making design improvements on the basis of the result, and then repeating the analyses or tests again, followed by further design improvements. This case entailed several design iterations of the VHR medication kit. The final version was tested with new recruits who, without training, were able to navigate the kit efficiently and without errors.

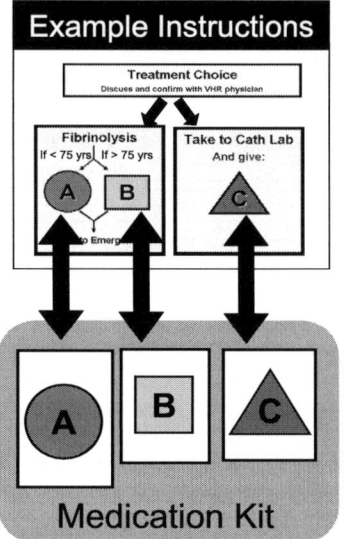

Figure 10-4. Example of Instruction with Mapping of Graphical Information to Medication Kit Layout

This illustration shows how graphical information in instructions can be mapped to the physical layout of a medication kit. Boxes A, B, and C in the medication kit each contain different combinations and doses of medications. A color version of this figure is also provided online (http:/www.jcrinc.com/UHFE10/extras).

Source: ISMP Canada. Used with permission.

The VHR team also took information from the two nonfatal incidents and translated that into design changes that would provide a more robust and permanent safeguard against similar incidents in the future. The design improvements reduced the mental burden on paramedics and improved the efficiency of the protocol.

In summary, we used various human factors principles and concepts to make changes to the VHR medication kit. Other human factors issues identified were centered around other devices or products, such as the communication and electrocardiograph transmission system, medication packaging and labeling, medication delivery devices, hospital forms, and medication supply and expiration date control. Although the VHR team did not have much control over the design of these devices or products, they could use the information for future procurement decisions.

Case Study 5. Forensic Usability Test for Ambulatory Infusion Pump and Chemotherapy Intravenous Bag Label

In 2006 a 43-year-old woman received an infusion of 5-fluorouracil (5-FU) in four hours instead of the four days as prescribed at a large cancer center. The inadvertent overdose resulted in the patient's death. The cancer center invited ISMP Canada to undertake a root cause analysis (RCA) of this event. RCA is a structured process that reviews an event with the goals of determining what happened, identifying the causes of the event, and translating the identified causes into redesign to reduce the likelihood of a recurrence. In brief, the RCA involved several dozen hours per person in on-site observation and interviewing, as well as post hoc analysis of the data and other expert resources. The full RCA report was made available to the public.[8]

ISMP Canada contracted with an HFE consultant to provide additional HFE analysis, including a forensic usability test of the infusion pump and associated materials (for example, chemotherapy IV bag). On-site evaluation of work tools and processes were needed to prepare the protocol for the usability test. The test itself was conducted at another cancer center unfamiliar with the infusion pump and ignorant of the case.

Task Analysis (Preparation for Usability Test)

The HFE consultant, together with the RCA team lead (from ISMP Canada), conducted several interviews with nurses, pharmacists, and biomedical engineers with knowledge about the process and tools. They then observed the steps needed to attach a 5-FU IV bag and infusion pump to a patient in an infusion-center setting. Initially, the following four items were gathered together on a countertop:

1. Ambulatory infusion pump (approximately the size and appearance of a handheld video game controller)
2. Labeled IV bag with attached tubing
3. Handheld calculator
4. Paper chart and medication administration record (MAR) sheet for documentation of administration

Protocol for Usability Test

The overall approach was that of a usability test, with the focus on task completion and errors (if any) and not on the time taken to complete the task.[9] The number of participants was in accord with both the scope and resources of the overall project in mind and with an estimate of how confusing the pump and chemotherapy label would likely be.

Five nurses, each with a special oncology nursing degree and more than five years' experience in working in oncology settings, volunteered to assist with the usability test. All had many years of experience in working with ambulatory infusion pumps (but not this particular brand) in ambulatory infusion settings. The stated goal of the usability test was to simulate use of the pump and IV bag label to contribute to their redesign. The pump, IV bag with label, calculator, pad of paper, and pen were arranged as was done at the cancer clinic at which the incident occurred.

The scenario was explained in the following manner: (a) the patient was in a chair at the clinic; (b) the chart had already been reviewed, with proper laboratory values and the medication information on the bag label confirmed; and (c) the nurse had now come back to his or her work area to program and assemble the pump.

The participants were told that they could think out loud or comment but that they would not be reminded or interrupted after they began. The following data were collected through observation:
1. Correct and incorrect steps taken to power on, assemble, program, and activate the pump
2. Questions asked or major confusion with any of the steps
3. Less efficient but ultimately workable pathways taken to program the pump
4. How the pump was programmed

The test director/observer also played the role of another nurse, who could be asked questions about this "new" pump and for double-checking programming.

Summary of Findings
The findings of the usability test were as follows:
1. One participant replicated all aspects of the incorrect infusion pump programming and three replicated some aspects.
2. All five participants were confused with one or more aspects of powering on, setting up, and selection of "mL/hr" choice for programming the pump.
3. One of the five participants noted that other IV bag labels in her job are laid out (organized) according to the sequence and terminology to be followed for the pump being used. She found it disconcerting that this was not the case here.
4. Three of the five participants commented on one or more design aspects of the pump or the IV bag label. Interestingly, the two participants who had some confusion with programming had no negative comments (complaints) about the design. This is not surprising, given that health care personnel often work around poor design with little complaint.

Recommendations
Findings from the usability testing informed the recommendations made in the final RCA report, which addressed optimal labeling and display of information; mapping (matching) the sequence and terms used for medication-associated values among electronic and printed documents (for example, MAR, bag, IV pump); training; and selection of ambulatory infusion pumps.

SUMMARY
ISMP Canada continues to integrate human factors expertise into its work. The value of balancing professional clinical input with technical expertise to improve medication safety design is becoming more widely recognized. How a medication is packaged, stocked, dispensed, and administered; its color and shape; and how it works with other components or parts of the system, including the various technologies—all these elements can be engineered for safety. Designing or redesigning a medication system to prevent or reduce medication errors requires

CHAPTER 10
Integrating Human Factors Engineering into Medication Safety at ISMP Canada

the perspective of people who understand the context in which medications or devices are used (that is, practical experience), and an understanding of how people interact with their environments (that is, psychology and engineering). The integration of the varied areas of expertise and the collaborative approach to identified problems and provided an opportunity for synergy as we work to improve medication safety in health care organizations.

The authors express their sincere appreciation to the many health care professionals who have demonstrated support for a culture of safety, exemplified by their willingness to share information about medication incidents and related findings. Case Study 4. Emergency Medical Service Medication Kit was kindly provided by Laura Lin Gosbee, M.A.Sc. (Donna Walsh, R.N., was the ISMP Canada team lead), and reviewed by Darren Knapp, Jessica Deckert-Sookram, and Shelley Valaire of Alberta Health Services. Case Study 5. Forensic Usability Test for Ambulatory Infusion Pump and Chemotherapy Intravenous Bag Label was kindly provided by John W. Gosbee, M.D., M.S. (ISMP Canada staff member Julie Greenall was the root cause analysis team lead). The authors also gratefully acknowledge manuscript advice from David K. U, R.Ph., M.Sc.Phm., President and CEO of ISMP Canada, and editorial review of the chapter by Corinne Hodgson.

References

1. Institute for Safe Medication Practices (ISMP) Canada: *Home Page.* http://www.ismp-canada.org/index.htm (accessed Apr. 2, 2010).
2. Institute for Safe Medication Practices (ISMP): *Home Page.* http://www.ismp.org/ (accessed Apr. 2, 2010).
3. Health Canada: *Canadian Medication Incident Reporting and Prevention System (CMIRPS).* http://www.hc-sc.gc.ca/dhp-mps/pubs/medeff/_fs-if/2004-cmirps-scdpim/ (accessed Apr. 2, 2010).
4. ISMP Canada: Sentinel event with sterile water—Lessons shared. *ISMP Canada Safety Bulletin* 2:4, Apr. 2002.
5. ISMP Canada: Enhanced sterile water label paves way for national standard. *ISMP Canada Safety Bulletin* 3:1–2, Jun. 6, 2003. http://www.ismp-canada.org/download/safetyBulletins/ISMPCSB2003-06SterileWater.pdf (accessed Apr. 2, 2010).
6. Greenall J., et al.: Medication safety alerts. *Canadian Journal of Hospital Pharmacy* 58:110–113, Apr. 2004. http://www.ismp-canada.org/download/cjhp/cjhp0404.pdf (accessed Apr. 5, 2010).
7. Institute for Safe Medication Practices (ISMP) Canada: *Failure Mode and Effects Analysis (FMEA).* http://www.ismp-canada.org/fmea.htm (accessed Apr. 2, 2010).
8. Institute for Safe Medication Practices Canada: *Fluorouracil Incident Root Cause Analysis,* May 22, 2007. http://www.cancerboard.ab.ca/NR/rdonlyres/2FB61BC4-70CA-4E58-BDE1-1E54797BA47D/0/FluorouracilIncidentMay2007.pdf (accessed Apr. 5, 2010).
9. Dumas J.S., Redish J.C.: *A Practical Guide to Usability Testing, rev. ed.* London: Intellect, 1999.

Index

A

AAMI (Association for Advancement of Medical Instrumentation), 38, 72
ACM (Association for Computing Machinery), 74
Admission forms and process, 129–130, 131
Advocate Christ Medical Center CHF order sets design, 5, 52
Air temperature, 27–28
Alarms or auditory feedback. *See also* Hearing and sounds
    "failure to respond" problem, solution to, 105–108, 109, 136
    intensity variations, 14, 15
    noise and, 27, 38
    redundant cues, 19
    sound localization, 15
Alberta Health Services (Capital Health Region), 150–153
American National Standards Institute (ANSI), 38, 72
Ames room, 12, 13
Analysis methods and tools, 36, 37, 38–41, 46. *See also Specific methods and tools*
Anchoring on initial hypothesis, 17
Anesthesia Patient Safety Foundation, 81
Anesthesiology
    anesthesia machines, 15, 43, 81, 135
    patient safety and HFE, 135–137
ANSI (American National Standards Institute), 38, 72
Anthropometric tables, 22, 23–24
Artifact model, 40
Association for Advancement of Medical Instrumentation (AAMI), 38, 72
Association for Computing Machinery (ACM), 74
Attention. *See* Memory and attention
Automatic behavior, 20
Average person, 21
Aviation industry, 4, 82–83

B

Barnes-Jewish Hospital, 118, 120–134
Baylor Health Care System HFE and patient safety research, 79–80, 137–142
    electronic health records, implementation of, 139–141, 142
    HFE professionals, recruitment and role of, 137–139
    patient education on self-care skills, 141–142
Bed monitors, 22
Binocular disparity (stereopsis), 12
Biomedical engineering department, 139
BJC HealthCare patient safety and quality program, 79, 117–134
    admission forms and process, 130, 131
    BJC WellAware employee health program, 118–119
    Center for Healthcare Quality and Effectiveness (Center for Clinical Excellence), 120
    discharge process, 120, 130, 131
    ED admission process, 129–130, 131
    human factors module, 120–121, 122
    inpatient medical processes improvements, 128–130, 131
    medical equipment availability improvement initiative, 121–128
    nitrogen oxide and carbon dioxide tube connection errors, 130–131, 132, 133
    plan of care transparency, 130, 131
Blame and shame/blame and train attitude, 4, 35–36, 82
Body temperature, 24–25
Bottom-up processing, 15
Bradycardia algorithm, 64
Breaks, frequency and length of, 25
Brightness (luminance), 26

C

Calcium gluconate, 147–148
Canadian Institute for Health Information, 145
Canadian Medication Incident Reporting and Prevention System, 145
Cancer treatment
   coupling of systems in cancer centers, 31
   ISMP Canada infusion pump and IV bag usability test, 153–154
Capital Health Region (Alberta Health Services), 150–153
Cardiac monitoring, 84–85
Carpal tunnel syndrome, 7
Case studies and examples
   Advocate Christ Medical Center CHF order sets design, 5, 52
   Baylor Health Care System HFE and patient safety research, 79–80, 137–142
      electronic health records, implementation of, 139–141, 142
      HFE professionals, recruitment and role of, 137–139
      patient education on self-care skills, 141–142
   BJC HealthCare patient safety and quality program, 79, 117–134
      admission forms and process, 130, 131
      BJC WellAware employee health program, 118–119
      Center for Healthcare Quality and Effectiveness (Center for Clinical Excellence), 120
      discharge process, 120, 130, 131
      ED admission process, 129–130, 131
      human factors module, 120–121, 122
      inpatient medical processes improvements, 128–130, 131
      medical equipment availability improvement initiative, 121–128
      nitrogen oxide and carbon dioxide tube connection errors, 130–131, 132, 133
      plan of care transparency, 130, 131
   Institute for Safe Medication Practices Canada (ISMP Canada) HFE integration and medication safety, 80, 145–155
   Johns Hopkins Hospital HFE and patient safety, 79, 103–115
      alarm management, 105–108, 109
      equipment supply project, 108–113
   Kent Hospital HFE response to patient-safety issues, 83–88
   St. Mark's Hospital code cart design, 49–52
   Sunnybrook and Women's Health Sciences Center epinephrine auto-injector exercise, 46, 47
   Sunnybrook Health Sciences Centre patient safety service, 79, 89–102
      CPOE system, 99–101
      critical care clinical information system, 97–99
      Human Factors 101 course, 91–92, 94–95
      smart infusion pump evaluation, 92–93, 96–97, 102
   University of Toronto PCA pump investigation, 46–49
Cause-and-effect matrix, 129
Central lines, 83, 136
Chapanis, Alphonse, 103
Chemotherapy IV bags, 153–154
Chest tubes, 136
Chunks of information, 16
Circadian rhythms, 24–25
Climate, 27–28, 30, 31
Clinical information system
   analysis and evaluation of, 138–139
   clinical practice guidelines, 5
   contextual inquiry and usability of, 41
   critical care clinical information system, 97–99
   emergency scenario reminder cards, 64
Clinical decision support systems
   Failure Mode and Effects Analysis, 138
Clinical practice guidelines, 5
Clinicians
   autonomy of physicians, 82
   communication between HFE professional and, 142
   HFE professionals, former clinicians as, 68–69
   teaching HFE mind-set and practice to, 57, 61, 62, 64–65, 138
Code cart design, 4, 41, 49–52
Code resources, 16
Cognitive capabilities and limitations
   cognitive tunnel vision, 17
   designing systems to accommodate limitations, 7, 18–21

INDEX

folk models on, 141
human information processing model, 7–8, 10–11
Cognitive map, 17
Cognitive task analysis, 39, 47, 140, 142
Cognitive tunnel vision, 17
Cognitive walk-through, 151
Cognitive work analysis, 37, 39–40
Communication
    ED admission process and, 129–130, 131
    between HFE professional and health care provider, 142
    noise and, 27
Complexity
    HFE and, v
    medical equipment and, v, 3
    product design and, 3
    of systems, v, 29, 31
Computerized order entry
    Failure Mode and Effects Analysis, 138
Computerized physician order entry (CPOE) system
    analysis and evaluation of, 138–139
    design of, 36, 38
    mortality rate and, 140
    task analysis and, 39
    usability testing, 99–101
Computerized Provider Order Entry (CPOE) systems
    case study, 99–101
Computers
    human-computer interaction (HCI) design, 20–21, 55–56
    human-computer interaction (HCI) resources, 74–75
    for patient and family education, 138
    scenario-based evaluation methodologies, 138
    usability testing, 41
Confirmation bias, 17
Congestive heart failure (CHF)
    mortality and readmission rates, 141, 142
    order sets design, 5, 52, 63–64
Consistency
    automatic behavior and, 20
    HCI design and, 21
Contextual inquiry, 40–41, 42
Contrast dye for imaging study, 83
Contrast sensitivity, 5, 11–12

Coupling, 29, 31
Crash cart medication drawer design, 4, 41, 46, 49–52
Crew resource management (CRM), 82–83
Critical care clinical information system, 97–99
CRM (crew resource management), 82–83
Cultural model, 40

D

Data collection
    system analysis and, 36
    task analysis, 38–39
Decision making
    biases in, 17–18
    information processing and, 10
    process for, 18
    stages of, 17
Defense, U.S. Department of, 73, 74
Defibrillator/pacemaker, 19
Depth and size perception, 12, 13
Discharge process, 120, 130, 131
Discriminability, 19
Displays
    definition of, 18
    design of, 18–20, 38, 61, 63, 64
    vibration and, 28
Divided attention, 16, 19–20
Drug-delivery system, design of, 43

E

ECRI/ECRI Institute, 5, 74, 105
Edmonton EMS, 150–153
Education and training
    blame and train attitude, 4, 35–36, 82
    contextual inquiry and learning processes and tools, 41, 42
    of HFE professionals, v, 67–68, 69
    Human Factors 101 course, 91–92, 94–95
    human factors module, 120–121, 122
    learning, long-term memory and, 17
    on medical equipment use, 3, 38
    patient and family education, computers for, 138
    patient education on self-care skills, 141–142
    patient safety curriculum development, 59
    in research methodology, 70
    resources, 71
    teaching HFE mind-set and practice, 57, 59

to clinicians, 57, 61, 62, 64–65, 138
to leadership, 57, 59, 61, 63–64, 71
to medical students and trainees, 59–60
pearls of teaching HFE, 64–65
simulation as teaching tool, 46
usability testing as teaching tool, 46, 47
workshop objectives and agendas, 59, 60, 61, 62
usability testing and design of training materials, 41, 43
Electronic health records
design flaws, 139, 141
design of, v
errors associated with, 139, 140, 141
hazard analysis of, 140–141
implementation of, 139–141, 142
Electronic order entry system
design of, v
proximity compatibility and, 19
working memory and, 20
Electrosurgical devices, 22
Emergency department (ED)
admission process, 129–130
critical care clinical information system, 97–99
Kent Hospital HFE response to patient-safety issues, 79, 84–88
redesign of, 84, 86–88
Emergency medical services medication kits, 150–153
Emergency medical technicians, 28
Emergency medical transportation
climate and, 28
noise and, 27
vibration and, 28
Emergency scenario reminder cards, 64
Employee health program, 117, 118–119
End users, 41
Engineering psychology, 4
Environmental factors
climate, 27–28, 30, 31
illumination, 25–26, 30, 89
noise, 26–27, 30, 38
vibration, 28–29, 31
Epinephrine auto-injectors, 19, 46, 47, 57
Ergonomics
computer placement and, 138
definition of, 4
employee health program, 118, 119

importance of, 22
purpose of, 4
research on, 22
Errors and adverse events
blame and shame/blame and train attitude, 4, 35–36, 82
coupling of systems and, 31
CPOE system and, 140
data collection, system analysis and, 36
design of systems and, 4–5, 35–36
EHRs and, 139, 140, 141
exercise to identify HFE issues, 8, 9
HFE approach to response to, 132, 133–134
medication-related events
Canadian Medication Incident Reporting and Prevention System, 145
culture of blame, 146
designing and redesigning systems to prevent, 154–155
exercise to identify HFE issues, 8, 9
ISMP Canada focus and mission, 145–146
nitrogen oxide and carbon dioxide tube connection errors, 130–131, 132, 133
reactive approach to, 83
system failures behind, 4
Errors and error messages, HCI design and, 21
Exercises
Gaining Insight, 6
HFE issues in Medication Administration, 8, 9
Practice Observing HFE issues, 7
Eyewear, protective, 82

F

FAA (Federal Aviation Administration), 73, 74
Failure Mode and Effects Analysis (FMEA)
identification of hazards with, 45–46, 105, 113, 129, 138
steps in, 150
sterile water labeling change analysis, 150
Failure mode causes, 45, 46
Fatigue and sleep deprivation, 22, 24–25
Fault tree analysis, 105–108, 113
Feasibility analysis, 113–114
Federal Aviation Administration (FAA), 73, 74
Feedback, HCI design and, 21
Fentanyl transdermal patches, 146–147
Figure-ground perception, 15
5S (sort, set in order, shine, standardize, sustain)

INDEX

technique, 123–124, 128
Flashlights, 89
Flooring materials and shoes, 119
Flow model, 40
FMEA. *See* Failure mode and effects analysis (FMEA)
Food and Drug Administration, U.S., 5, 72
Function analysis, 104

G

Gaining Insight exercise, 6
Glucometers, 43, 57

H

Hand-arm vibration, 28–29, 31
Hazard analysis, 140–141
Health Canada, 145
Health care organizations, HFE role in, 5, 81–82
Hearing and sounds
  damage to hearing, 26
  discrimination threshold, 14
  ear protection, 27
  HFE guideline examples, 19
  intensity discrimination, 14
  intensity variations, 14, 15
  interaural intensity differences, 15
  interaural time difference, 15
  loudness, 14, 26
  maximum noise levels, 27
  noise, 26–27
  range of hearing, 12, 14
  sound localization, 14–15
  sound shadow, 15
  threshold intensity, 12, 14
Heuristic evaluation
  example of, 58
  HFE issues identification, 37, 40, 56–57
  PCA pump evaluation, 47
  popularity of, 40
Human-computer interaction (HCI) design, 20–21, 55–56
Human-computer interaction (HCI) resources, 74–75
Human engineering, 4
Human Factors 101 course, 91–92, 94–95
Human Factors and Ergonomics Society, 68, 75
Human factors engineering (HFE)
  analysis methods and tools, 36, 37, 38–41, 46

  (*see also specific methods and tools*)
  attributes of, v
  complexity and, v
  concept of, v, 3–4
  design guidance, 36, 37, 38
    memory and attention, 19–20
    perception, 19
    physical limits and anthropometrics, 30–31
  leadership support for, 85–86
  learning, 5
  pearls of conducting HFE practice, 56–57
  recognition of, 6, 7, 32
  resources, 71–75
  role in everyday life, 81
  role in health care, 5, 81–82
  specialty areas, 74
  synonymous terms for, 4
Human factors engineering (HFE) professional
  assistance provided by, v, 91
  communication between health care providers and, 142
  cross-training of, 68–69
  education and training of, v, 67–68, 69
  finding, 91
  hiring tips, 68–70
  at Johns Hopkins Hospital, 103–115
  passion of, 70
  recruitment and role of, 137–139
Human users
  cognitive capabilities and limitations
    cognitive tunnel vision, 17
    designing systems to accommodate limitations, 7, 18–21
    human information processing model, 7–8, 10–11
  decision making
    biases in, 17–18
    information processing and, 10
    process for, 18
    stages of, 17
  limitations of, 5
  memory and attention
    automatic behavior, consistency, and, 20
    capabilities and limitations, 5
    divided attention, 16, 19–20
    expectancy and, 15
    HFE guideline examples, 19–20
    information processing and, 10

161

long-term memory, 17, 20
mental models, 17, 19
primacy effect, 17
saliency and, 15, 17
selective attention, 15–16
working memory, 16–18, 20, 141
perception
  bottom-up processing, 15
  contrast sensitivity, 5, 11–12, 19
  depth and size perception, 12, 13
  hearing, 12, 14–15
  HFE guideline examples, 19
  information processing and, 10
  pre-attentive processing, 15
  sensory processing, 10, 11–15
  top-down processing, 15
  vision, 5, 11–12, 13, 19, 104
physical limits and anthropometrics
  anthropometric tables, 22, 23–24
  average person, 21
  capabilities and limitations, 5, 7
  comfort for operator and system design, 36–37
  designing systems to accommodate limitations, 21–22
  environmental factors and, 25–29
  fatigue and sleep deprivation, 22, 24–25
  HFE guideline examples, 30–31
  posture and movement, 22, 25, 30
  work-arounds development, 3
Humidity levels, 27, 30

I

Illumination, 25–26, 30, 89
Impact matrix, 129
Information processing
  bottom-up processing, 15
  chunks of information, 16
  model, 7–8, 10–11
  pre-attentive processing, 15
  top-down processing, 15
Infusion pumps
  case studies and examples
    BJC HealthCare medical equipment availability improvement initiative, 121
    ISMP Canada infusion pump and IV bag usability test, 153–154
    Sunnybrook Health Sciences Centre evaluation of pumps, 92–93, 96–97, 102
  design of, v, 38
  heuristic evaluation and design of, 40
  illumination and programming of pumps, 89
Inhalers, 43
Injury-prevention program, 117, 118–119
Inpatient medical processes improvements, 128–130, 131
in situ simulation, 43
Institute for Safe Medication Practices (ISMP), 145, 146
Institute for Safe Medication Practices Canada (ISMP Canada)
  collaborative relationships with strategic partners, 145
  creation of, 145
  focus and mission of, 145–146
  HFE integration and medication safety, 80, 145–155
    calcium gluconate, 147–148
    emergency medical services medication kits, 150–153
    fentanyl transdermal patches, 146–147
    infusion pump and IV bag usability test, 153–154
    sterile water, 148–150
Institute of Medicine (IOM), *To Err is Human*, 81, 142
Insulin-injection pen display, 61, 63, 64
Intensive care units (ICUs). *See also* Neonatal intensive care units (NICUs)
  critical care clinical information system, 97–99
  pediatric intensive care units, 136
  posture and movement and design of, 22
Interaural intensity differences, 15
Interaural time difference, 15
International Ergonomics Association, 4, 75
International Standardization Organization (ISO), 72
Internet resources, 74–75
Intravenous medications
  ISMP Canada infusion pump and IV bag usability test, 153–154
  sterile water, 148–150
ISMP (Institute for Safe Medication Practices), 145, 146
ISMP Canada. *See* Institute for Safe Medication Practices Canada (ISMP Canada)

INDEX

ISO (International Standardization Organization), 72
Iterative design, 38, 40, 152–153

J

Jet lag, 24–25
Job and task design, 29, 31–32
Johns Hopkins Hospital HFE and patient safety, 79, 103–115
    alarm management, 105–108, 109
    equipment supply project, 108–113
Joint Commission, The, 75
Joint Commission Center for Transforming Healthcare, 75
Joint Commission International, 75
Just-in-time management philosophy, 31

K

Kent Hospital HFE response to patient-safety issues, 79, 83–88
Knowledge-based decision making, 18

L

Language, HCI design and, 20
Laparoscopic surgery
    laparoscopy equipment, 15, 22
    task analysis and, 39
Leadership
    support for HFE approach, 85–86
    teaching HFE mind-set and practice to, 57, 59, 61, 63–64, 71
Lean, 67, 118
Lean Six Sigma, 79, 120, 121, 123, 128, 132–133
Learning
    contextual inquiry and learning processes and tools, 41, 42
    HFE approach, 5
    long-term memory and, 17
Light intensity, 25–26, 30, 89
Link analysis, 129
Long-term memory, 17, 20
Loosely-coupled systems, 31
Luminance (brightness), 26

M

Magazines and journals, 73
Magnet award, 86
Marquette University, Rehabilitation Engineering Center on Accessible Medical Instrumentation, 75

Medical devices and equipment
    alarms or auditory feedback
        "failure to respond" problem, solution to, 105–108, 109, 136
        intensity variations, 14, 15
        noise and, 27, 38
        redundant cues, 19
        sound localization, 15
    analysis and user testing of, 37
    case studies and examples
        BJC HealthCare medical equipment availability improvement initiative, 121–128
        Johns Hopkins Hospital equipment supply project, 108–113
        Sunnybrook Health Sciences Centre usability testing, 92—93, 96–97
    cleaning process, 121–128
    climate and, 28
    complexity and, v, 3
    heuristic evaluation example, 58
    HFE and development of, 5
    identification of HFE issues, 56–57, 61, 63, 64
    lighting and, 26
    noise and, 27
    pre-attentive processing, design for, 15
    RCA and design solutions, 45–46
    redundant cues, 19
    training to use, 3, 38
    usability data and procurement decisions, 45
    usability testing and procurement decisions, 43, 44, 45, 63, 93, 96–102
    usability testing as teaching tool, 46
Medical gases tube connection errors, 130–131, 132, 133
Medical processes improvements, 128–130, 131
Medical students and residents
    contextual inquiry and learning processes and tools, 41, 42
    epinephrine auto-injector exercise, 46, 47
    teaching HFE mind-set and practice to, 59–60
Medications
    complexity and processes associated with, 3
    discriminability and drug names, 19
    divided attention and, 16
    drug-delivery system, design of, 43
    errors and adverse events
        Canadian Medication Incident Reporting and Prevention System, 145

culture of blame, 146
designing and redesigning systems to prevent, 154–155
exercise to identify HFE issues, 8, 9
ISMP Canada focus and mission, 145–146
HFE issues in Medication Administration exercise, 8, 9
labeling changes, 149–150
medication incident, definition of, 145
medication reconciliation process, 129, 131
medication safety and HFE, 146–155
    calcium gluconate, 147–148
    emergency medical services medication kits, 150–153
    fentanyl transdermal patches, 146–147
    infusion pump and IV bag usability test, 153–154
    sterile water, 148–150
narcotics cabinets, design of, 22
redundant cues, 149–150
storage areas, design of, 22
Memory and attention
    automatic behavior, consistency, and, 20
    capabilities and limitations, 5
    divided attention, 16, 19–20
    expectancy and, 15
    HFE guideline examples, 19–20
    information processing and, 10
    long-term memory, 17, 20
    mental models, 17, 19
    primacy effect, 17
    saliency and, 15, 17
    selective attention, 15–16
    working memory, 16–18, 20, 141
Mental models, 17, 19
Mental simulation, 18
Michael J. Woods Institute, 84, 86
Miriam Hospital, The, 82–83
Modality resources, 16
Mortality rates, 140, 141
Motion parallax, 12, 13
Movement and posture, 22, 25, 30
Multidisciplinary Assessment of Technology Centre for Health Care (MATCH), 37–38
Multiple resource theory, 16
Muscular effort, 25
Muscular exhaustion, 25

N

Narcotics cabinets, design of, 22
National Center for Patient Safety (NCPS), 90
NCPS (National Center for Patient Safety), 90
Neonatal intensive care units (NICUs)
    cognitive task analysis and, 39
    cognitive work analysis and, 39
    Vermont Oxford Network NICQ project, 92
Nitrogen oxide and carbon dioxide tube connection errors, 130–131, 132, 133
Noise, 26–27, 30, 38
Nuclear power industry, 4
Nuclear Regulatory Commission, U.S., 73
Nurses. See Clinicians

O

Observing HFE issues exercise, 7
Ontario Neurotrauma Foundation, 119
Ontario Safety Association for Community and Healthcare (OSACH), 119
Operating rooms and theaters. See also Surgical procedures
    anesthesiology
        anesthesia machines, 15, 43, 81, 135
        patient safety and HFE, 135–137
    checklist use in, 82
    cognitive work analysis and, 39–40
    drug-delivery system, design of, 43
    Johns Hopkins Hospital equipment supply project, 108–113
    lighting in, 26
    nitrogen oxide and carbon dioxide tube connection errors, 130–131, 132, 133
    posture and movement and design of, 22
    sociotechnical system to coordinate activities in, 136
    sound localization and, 15
    work flow in, 137
Order forms. See also Computerized physician order entry (CPOE) system; Electronic order entry system
    CHF order sets, 4, 52
    design of, 36, 63–64
Organizational structure, 29, 31
OSACH (Ontario Safety Association for Community and Healthcare), 119

INDEX

P

Patient and family education, computers for, 138
Patient-controlled analgesia (PCA) pumps
    cognitive task analysis of, 47
    errors with and HFE design issues, 35–36
    heuristic evaluation of, 40, 47
    human factors study of, 46–49
    Johns Hopkins Hospital color-coding on pumps, 104
    redesign of, 47–49
    University of Toronto PCA pump investigation, 46–49
    working memory and settings on, 16–17
Patient education on self-care skills, 141–142
Patient identification, 89, 130, 139
Patient lifting and moving, 22, 30, 118
Patient safety
    blame and shame/blame and train attitude, 4, 35–36, 82
    curriculum development for medical schools and teaching hospitals, 59
    HFE approach to, 4, 5, 83, 113–115
    HFE techniques and, 44–46
Pearls of conducting HFE practice, 56–57
Pearls of teaching HFE, 64–65
Pediatric intensive care units, 136
Perception
    bottom-up processing, 15
    contrast sensitivity, 5, 11–12, 19
    depth and size perception, 12, 13
    hearing, 12, 14–15
    HFE guideline examples, 19
    information processing and, 10
    pre-attentive processing, 15
    sensory processing, 10, 11–15
    top-down processing, 15
    vision, 5, 11–12, 13, 19, 104
Peripherally inserted central catheter (PICC) line, 83
Pharmacy systems and HFE issues, 55–56
Physical limits and anthropometrics
    anthropometric tables, 22, 23–24
    average person, 21
    capabilities and limitations, 5, 7
    comfort for operator and system design, 36–37
    designing systems to accommodate limitations, 21–22
    environmental factors and, 25–29
    fatigue and sleep deprivation, 22, 24–25
    HFE guideline examples, 30–31
    posture and movement, 22, 25, 30
Physical model, 40
Physicians. *See* Clinicians
PICC (peripherally inserted central catheter) line, 83
Plan-Do-Check-Act cycle, 119
Plan of care transparency, 130, 131
Posture and movement, 22, 25, 30
Practice Observing HFE issues exercise, 7
Pre-attentive processing, 15
Primacy effect, 17
Processing stage resources, 16
Project management, 133
Proximity compatibility principle, 19

R

Radiation treatment, 3
Rational process tools, 133
Readmission rates, 141, 142
Recognition-primed decision making, 18
Redundant cues, 19, 149–150
Repetitive movements, 25
Research methodology, 70
Resources, 71–75
Resuscitation units, 136
Return on investment (ROI), 85, 86
Root cause analysis (RCA)
    actions or solutions based on, 45–46, 61, 82
    heuristic evaluation and, 40
    investigation of error with, 35, 45, 61, 153
Rule-based decision making, 18

S

St. Mark's Hospital code cart design, 4, 41, 46, 49–52
Salient cues, 15, 17
Scenario-based evaluation methodologies, 138
Schema, 17
SEIPS (Systems Engineering Initiative for Patient Safety), 119–120
Selective attention, 15–16
Sensory processing, 10, 11–15
Sequence model, 40
Shift work, 24–25
Shoes and flooring materials, 119

Shortcuts, 21
Short-term memory, 16–17
Simulation or simulator testing
    HFE issues identification with, 37, 41, 43
    PCA pump redesign testing, 47–48
    as teaching tool, 46
Single resource theory, 16
Six Sigma, 67, 79, 117, 120–121, 123, 132–133
Size and depth perception, 12, 13
Skill-based decision making, 18
Sleep deprivation and fatigue, 22, 24–25
Software
    design of, v
    heuristic evaluation and design of, 40
    human-computer interaction (HCI) design, 20–21, 55–56
    identification of HFE issues, 57
    selective attention and design of, 15–16
Sort, set in order, shine, standardize, sustain (5S) technique, 123–124, 128
Sounds. See Hearing and sounds
Spatial code, 16
Specialty areas, 74
STEMI (ST-segment elevation myocardial infarction), 150–153
Stereopsis (binocular disparity), 12
Sterile water, 148–150
Storage areas, 22
Stove-top layout exercise, 61, 63
ST-segment elevation myocardial infarction (STEMI), 150–153
Sunnybrook and Women's Health Sciences Center epinephrine auto-injector exercise, 46, 47
Sunnybrook Health Sciences Centre patient safety service, 79, 89–102
    CPOE system, 99–101
    critical care clinical information system, 97–99
    Human Factors 101 course, 91–92, 94–95
    smart infusion pump evaluation, 92–93, 96–97, 102
Surgical procedures. See also Operating rooms and theaters
    electrosurgical devices, 22
    laparoscopic surgery
        laparoscopy equipment, 15, 22
        task analysis and, 39
    retained sponge RCA, 61
    wrong-site surgeries, 83

Syringes, discriminability and, 19
Systems and processes
    acceptance of, 36
    clumsy designs, v
    comfort for operator and, 36–37
    complexity of, v, 29, 31
    coupling of, 29, 31
    design of, v, 3
        art and science of, 36
        cognitive limitations, accommodation of, 7, 18–21
        error prevention, 154–155
        errors and, 4–5, 35–36
        Gaining Insight exercise, 6
        iterative design, 38, 40, 152–153
        Observing HFE issues exercise, 6
        patient safety and, 83
        RCA and design solutions, 45–46, 61
        user-centered design, 38
    effectiveness of, 36
    efficiency of, 36
    examples of, 3–4
    HFE design guidance, 36, 37, 38
        memory and attention, 19–20
        perception, 19
        physical limits and anthropometrics, 30–31
    identification of HFE issues, 56–57
    medical processes improvements, 128–130, 131
    system failures
        adverse events and, 4
        examples of, 4
Systems Engineering Initiative for Patient Safety (SEIPS), 119–120
Systems thinking, 70

T

Task analysis, 37, 38–39, 45, 104
Task and job design, 29, 31–32
Teaching HFE mind-set and practice. See Education and training
Temperature
    air temperature, 27–28
    body temperature, 24–25
Textural gradients, 12
Thoracostomy, HFE analysis of, 64–65, 136
Thoracostomy instruments, 136
Three-dimensional (3D) world, 12

Tightly-coupled systems, 31
To Err is Human (IOM), 81, 142
Top-down processing, 15
Training. *See* Education and training

U

Ultrasound system, 41
Umbrella sleeves, 119
University Health Network, 46, 74
University of Maryland School of Medicine, 135–136
University of Toronto
    engineering program, 91
    PCA pump investigation, 46–49
Usability engineering, 4
Usability testing
    code cart design, 49–52
    CPOE system evaluation, 99–101
    critical care clinical information system evaluation, 97–99
    focus and scope of, 37, 41, 43
    HFE issues identification with, 36, 37, 46
    infusion pump and IV bag usability test, 153–154
    iterative design and, 38
    procurement decisions and, 43, 44, 45, 63, 93, 96–102
    smart infusion pump evaluation, 92–93, 96–97, 102
    as teaching tool, 46, 47
User-centered design, 38
User testing, 37, 38, 41, 43

V

Value stream analysis, 120, 129, 130, 131
Ventilators
    operational failures, 43, 44
    usability testing and procurement decisions, 43
Verbal code, 16
Vermont Oxford Network NICQ project, 92
Veterans Affairs, Department of (VA), 90
VHR (Vital Heart Response) medication kits, 150–153
Vibration, 28–29, 31
Vision
    color-coding on PCA pumps, 104
    contrast sensitivity, 5, 11–12, 19
    depth and size perception, 12, 13
    HFE guideline examples, 19
Visual channel resources, 16
Vital Heart Response (VHR) medication kits, 150–153

W

Washington University School of Medicine, 118
White fingers, 7, 28, 31
Whole-body vibration, 28–29
Woods, James, 85
Woods, Michael J., 84–85
Work areas
    climate, 27–28, 30, 31
    HFE guideline examples, 30–31
    illumination, 25–26, 30, 89
    noise, 26–27, 30, 38
    vibration, 28–29, 31
Working memory, 16–18, 20, 141
Work-related injuries, 117, 118–119
Wrong-site surgeries, 83